Mayo Clinic on
Prostate Health

3rd EDITION

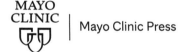

MAYO CLINIC | Mayo Clinic Press

MAYO CLINIC PRESS

Medical Editors | Derek J. Lomas, M.D.,
Paras H. Shah, M.D.
Publisher | Daniel J. Harke
Editor in Chief | Nina E. Wiener
Senior Editor | Karen R. Wallevand
Art Director | Stewart J. Koski
Production Design | Gunnar T. Soroos
Editorial Research Librarians | Anthony J. Cook, Edward
(Eddy) S. Morrow Jr., Erika A. Riggin, Katherine (Katie) J.
Warner, Morgan T. Wentworth
Contributors | Eugene D. Kwon, M.D., Heather LaBruna,
Ryan M. Phillips, M.D.
Image Credits | All photographs and illustrations are
copyright of Mayo Foundation for Medical Education
and Research (MFMER) except for the following:
NAME: GettyImages-1161154191.jpg/PAGE: Cover/
CREDIT: © Wavebreakmedia-iStock/Getty Images Plus

Additional contributions from Kirkus Reviews and Rath
Indexing

To stay informed about Mayo Clinic Press,
please subscribe to our free e-newsletter at
MCPress.MayoClinic.org or follow us on social media.

The information in this book is true and complete to the
best of our knowledge. This book is intended only as an
informative guide for those wishing to learn more about
health issues. It is not intended to replace, countermand
or conflict with advice given to you by your own
physician. The ultimate decision concerning your care
should be made between you and your doctor.
Information in this book is offered with no guarantees.
The authors and publisher disclaim all liability in
connection with the use of this book.

For bulk sales to employers, member groups and
health-related companies, contact Mayo Clinic,
200 First St. SW, Rochester, MN 55905, or email
SpecialSalesMayoBooks@mayo.edu.

ISBN 978-1-945564-09-3

Library of Congress Control Number: 2022935495

Printed in the United States of America

**When you purchase Mayo Clinic newsletters
and books, proceeds are used to further medical
education and research at Mayo Clinic. You not
only get answers to your questions on health,
you become part of the solution.**

Contents

Improving PSA testing
Answers to your questions

Cystoscopy
Ultrasound
X-ray
Computerized tomography (CT)
Magnetic resonance imaging (MRI)
MRI-ultrasound fusion
Nuclear scan
Bone scan
Positron emission tomography (PET)

Types of prostatitis
Diagnosing prostatitis
Treating prostatitis
Answers to your questions

A fact of life
Seeing a doctor
Next steps
Answers to your questions

Watchful waiting
Medications
Surgery

Minimally invasive surgical therapies
Transurethral surgery
Simple prostatectomy
Emerging treatments
Factors to consider
Answers to your questions

Signs and symptoms
Screening and diagnosis
Grading cancer
Biopsy tissue genomic testing
Additional tests
Cancer staging
What's next?
Answers to your questions

Taking stock
Active surveillance
Prostate cancer surgery
Radiation therapy
Focal therapy
Emerging treatments
Things to consider
Making your decision
Answers to your questions

Hormone therapy
Additional medications
Continuous versus intermittent therapy

Radiation and surgery
Relieving cancer pain
If your cancer returns
Answers to your questions

Managing incontinence
Managing erectile dysfunction
Other sexual concerns
Managing bowel disorders
Answers to your questions

Medical visits
Emotional toll
Regaining your strength
Eating better to feel better
Continuing to work
Communicating with others
Finding support
Answers to your questions

Potential cancer-fighting foods
A healthy diet
Physical activity
Seeing your doctor regularly
Answers to your questions

Preface

For some men, dealing with a prostate condition marks the first time they've visited a doctor in many years. Difficulties urinating — including frequent, urgent, weak or painful urination — become severe or disruptive enough that they decide it's time to seek medical care. Perhaps you're among this group.

Prostate problems are common. Most men experience a prostate condition at some point in their lives. The longer you live, the greater your odds of dealing with prostate enlargement, inflammation or cancer. The good news is these conditions can be successfully treated — even cancer. While prostate cancer remains the leading cause of cancer deaths in American men, great strides are being made in its diagnosis and treatment.

For cancer and other prostate conditions, advanced imaging technology allows doctors to identify prostate disease earlier, when the chances of successful treatment are greatest. And sophisticated medical procedures and therapies make it possible to treat prostate disease more specifically and precisely, improving the chances of a cure as well as reducing the risk of side effects.

The purpose of this book is to educate you about common prostate diseases, such as prostatitis, benign prostatic hyperplasia (BPH) and prostate cancer, and to empower you with knowledge that can help you ask the right questions and make informed decisions when faced with a prostate condition. You'll also find information on prostate screening tests and healthy behaviors and habits to improve prostate health.

The more you know about prostate disease, the greater your chances of identifying problems early, making good decisions about treatment and maintaining a high quality of life. The outlook for the management, cure and survival of prostate disease is better now than ever before.

Derek Lomas, M.D.
Paras Shah, M.D.

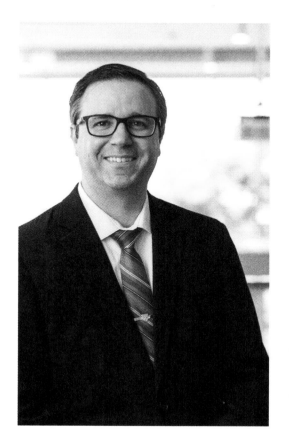

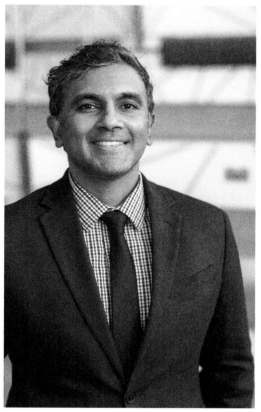

Derek J. Lomas, M.D., is a urologist at Mayo Clinic, Rochester, Minn. His clinical interests include prostate cancer diagnostics and imaging, focal therapies for the treatment of prostate cancer, and minimally invasive treatment of benign prostatic hyperplasia. Dr. Lomas received his residency training at Mayo Clinic, Rochester. He completed additional training as a Mayo Clinic Scholar at Imperial College London and University College London in the fields of prostate cancer imaging, targeted biopsy and focal therapy.

Paras H. Shah, M.D., is a urologic oncologist at Mayo Clinic, Rochester, Minn., specializing in the surgical management of prostate, bladder and kidney cancers with the use of robotic technology. Dr. Shah received his residency training at Long Island Jewish Medical Center, Queens, New York, and completed a fellowship in urologic oncology at Mayo Clinic, Rochester, Minn.

PART 1

Prostate basics

About the prostate gland

The prostate gland can cause some of the most common health problems that men face, and cancer of the prostate is among the most feared. That's because prostate cancer, like breast cancer for women, often strikes at the core of human sexuality.

Beyond the fear of cancer itself are the possible consequences of treatment — issues with bladder control (incontinence) or sexual complications, including erectile dysfunction, loss of ejaculation or changes in orgasm. These problems can be as difficult to deal with as the cancer, eroding your self-confidence and evoking feelings of lost masculinity.

But there's reason for optimism. If caught early, prostate cancer often can be successfully treated and cured. Improved

practices are reducing the risks of incontinence and erectile dysfunction. And when these complications do occur, treatment may limit their effects.

It's also important to understand that cancer isn't the only prostate problem. Inflammation and benign enlargement of the prostate are even more common developments. Unlike prostate cancer, these problems generally aren't life-threatening. But without proper treatment, they can become painful, and even debilitating.

Prostate problems are a fact of life for many men as they get older. However, with regular checkups, you can reduce your risk of serious disease and keep the condition from significantly disrupting your quality of life.

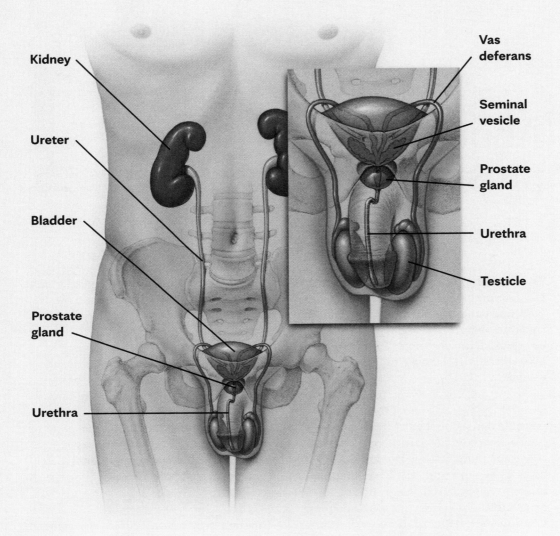

Kidney

Ureter

Bladder

Prostate
gland

Urethra

Vas
deferans

Seminal
vesicle

Prostate
gland

Urethra

Testicle

The prostate gland is tucked deep within the pelvic cavity, just below the bladder. Because of its location among so many organs, nerves, muscles and blood vessels, the prostate affects the health of both the reproductive system and urinary system.

This book can help you better understand why prostate problems occur, identify symptoms early and allow you to make informed decisions with your doctor regarding treatment.

A HEALTHY PROSTATE

Found only in men, the prostate gland lies at the base of the bladder. As urine drains from the bladder, it passes through the prostate.

At birth, the prostate is about the size of a pea. It continues to grow until about age 20, when it's roughly the size and shape of a walnut. The gland remains this size until your 40s, when it often starts to grow again. This second growth spurt is associated with prostate problems.

Treating prostate conditions can be difficult because the gland is bundled among many delicate organs, muscles, nerves and blood vessels. This is why side effects such as bleeding, incontinence and erectile dysfunction are always a concern — for example, prostate surgery may injure the nerves leading to the penis, causing erectile dysfunction.

Due to its location, the prostate gland plays a key role in the function of your reproductive system as well as your urinary system.

Reproductive system

Tiny glands in the prostate gland manufacture most of the fluid in semen. Ducts then carry this fluid to the urethra — the same channel that carries urine from the bladder out the penis.

During orgasm, prostate fluid mixes with fluid from the seminal vesicles, located on each side of the prostate, and with sperm to form semen. Sperm travel up from your testicles through long tubes called the vasa deferentia. Muscle contractions cause ejaculation, during which semen is propelled through the urethra and out the penis.

To make sure semen doesn't move in the wrong direction during ejaculation and back up into the bladder, a ring of muscle at the neck of the bladder, called the internal sphincter, tightens. The tightening closes the urethra. The internal sphincter also keeps urine from discharging with the semen.

Urinary system

Although the prostate gland isn't a primary component of the urinary system, it's important to urinary health.

Your urinary system begins with your kidneys, which cleanse body fluids and produce urine. Urine travels from your kidneys to your bladder through long muscular tubes called ureters. Your bladder stores the urine until you urinate. During urination, the bladder muscle contracts, and urine exits through the urethra and out the penis.

Your prostate gland surrounds the top portion of the urethra, just below the

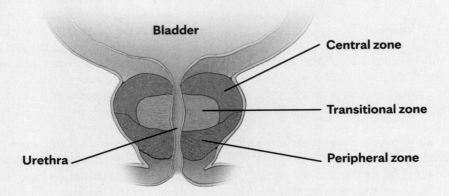

The prostate gland consists of smooth muscle and spongy tissue containing thousands of tiny glands and ducts. Two major types of cells make up the organ. Epithelial cells are found in the glands. They secrete the fluids used to produce semen — the fluid that transports and nourishes sperm. Stromal cells include connective tissue and smooth muscle that supports the epithelial cells.

The prostate also produces an enzyme known as prostate-specific antigen (PSA). This enzyme is vital in the reproductive process because it helps break down semen once the semen has been delivered to a woman's vagina, allowing the sperm to be freely mobile.

The prostate gland contains three sections (zones) that are separated by distinct structures and functions. The peripheral and central zones contain most of the prostate's glands, where semen fluid is produced. If prostate cancer develops, it's often in the peripheral zone, and then it spreads outward. The transitional zone, which surrounds the urethra in the center of the organ, is the part of your prostate that enlarges during the later growth stage that takes place in your 40s, exerting an inward pressure that can cause benign prostatic hyperplasia (BPH).

CROSS-SECTIONAL VIEW OF THE PELVIC ORGANS

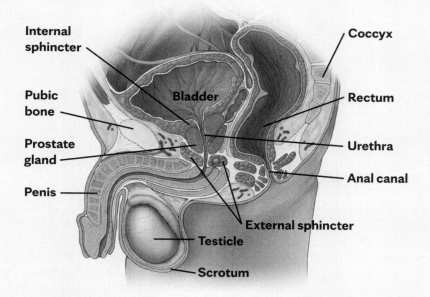

Internal sphincter

Pubic bone

Prostate gland

Penis

Bladder

Coccyx

Rectum

Urethra

Anal canal

External sphincter

Testicle

Scrotum

The prostate gland surrounds the upper portion of the urethra, a narrow canal that provides a passage for urine leaving the bladder and for semen used for reproduction.

bladder. Think of your prostate as a small apple with its core missing. The urethra runs through the missing core.

When the prostate is normal-size and healthy, the system functions properly. But disease can develop in the gland, causing tissue in the prostate to swell or grow. The swelling or growth squeezes the urethra, narrowing the drainage channel and affecting your ability to urinate.

WHEN THINGS GO WRONG

You aren't destined to develop prostate disease. Some men go through life without any prostate problems. Many, however, aren't so lucky. By the time they reach older adulthood, most men experience some type of prostate problem.

Symptoms of prostate disease may range from minor and mildly annoying to serious and painful.

Three different conditions commonly affect the prostate gland. Often, but not always, they can occur at different periods in a man's life.

Inflammation

Inflammation is the natural response of your body to infection or injury. Signs and symptoms often include redness, swelling and pain.

Your prostate gland can swell and become tender at any age. Often, a bacterial infection is the source of the inflammation. Other times, the cause of swelling and pain is unknown. Called prostatitis, prostate inflammation is the most common prostate problem among men under age 50.

Enlargement

Around age 45, tissue in your prostate gland often begins to grow again. This noncancerous growth is called benign prostatic hyperplasia (BPH). It typically occurs in the transitional zone — the central portion of the gland.

The growth typically moves inward, causing prostate tissue to squeeze against the urethra and produce urinary problems. It's the most common prostate problem for men ages 50 and older.

Cancer

According to the American Cancer Society, prostate cancer is the leading cause of cancer in American males. It most often occurs in men after age 50. The cancer results from abnormal and uncontrolled growth of tissue cells. Unlike BPH, cancerous tumors generally develop in the outer part of the prostate, particularly in the peripheral zone.

Depending on the specific makeup of the cancer, prostate tumors may grow very slowly or at a more rapid pace. The growth is generally outward, easily penetrating the thin membrane that encloses the prostate gland and spreading to surrounding tissue.

WARNING SIGNS

Irritation or pain will often alert you to prostate problems. This is especially true of prostate inflammation (prostatitis) or enlargement (BPH). Cancer typically provides less warning during its early stages.

The following signs and symptoms are often associated with prostate disease. However, they aren't limited to the prostate gland. Other conditions, such as a urinary infection, can produce similar signs and symptoms:

- Urinating more frequently.
- Excessive urination during the night (nocturia).
- Difficulty starting to urinate.
- Decreased force in urine stream.
- Interrupted flow of urine.
- Dribbling after finishing urination.
- Feeling as if your bladder isn't empty, even after urination.

ESTIMATED MALE CANCER CASES UNITED STATES, 2022

Total cases: 983,160

Cancer	Percent
Prostate	27%
Lung & bronchus	12%
Colon & rectum	8%
Urinary bladder	6%
Melanoma of skin	6%
Kidney & renal pelvis	5%
Non-Hodgkin's lymphoma	4%
Oral cavity & pharynx	4%
Leukemia	4%
Pancreas	3%
All other sites	21%

Data from American Cancer Society, 2022.

- Urgent need to urinate.
- Blood in your urine (hematuria).
- Pain or burning sensation while urinating (dysuria).
- Painful ejaculation.
- Tenderness or pain in the pelvis.
- Persistent back or hip pain.
- Pain or swelling in the testicles.

Unfortunately, prostate cancer produces few, if any, symptoms in its early stages. It's not until later, when the disease becomes more difficult to treat, that symptoms such as urinary difficulties or back pain may develop. That's why it's important to have regular prostate checkups to identify the disease early.

ARE YOU AT RISK?

There's no simple formula that predicts who will encounter prostate problems and at what point in life. However, various factors — some of which you can control — can affect your odds.

Uncontrollable factors

Factors that you can't control tend to be some of the most common risk factors of prostate disease.

Age

As you get older, your risk of both BPH and prostate cancer increases. It's estimated that about half the men in the United States between the ages of 51 and 60 and as many as 90% of men older than age 80 exhibit signs and symptoms of BPH. Indeed, it may be that all men will develop BPH if they live long enough.

The risk of prostate cancer also increases with age. About 60% of men diagnosed with prostate cancer are age 65 or older.

Race and ethnicity

In recent decades, prostate cancer death rates have dropped for all men, including Black men. However, Black men are more likely to get prostate cancer than men of other racial groups. They're also more likely to develop prostate cancer at a younger age and to develop an aggressive form of the disease. The reasons for this aren't well understood. Genetics, access to medical care, environment and lifestyle all may be factors.

According to the National Cancer Institute's Surveillance, Epidemiology, and End Results (SEER) database, Black men have overall prostate cancer mortality rates about twice as high as white, Hispanic and American Indian/Alaska Native men, and four times as high as Asian/Pacific Islander men. Asian/Pacific Islander men have the lowest rate of prostate cancer.

Because Black men are at higher risk of prostate cancer, some organizations advocate they begin prostate cancer screening earlier. The American Cancer Society recommends Black men discuss with their doctors the benefits and risks of starting screening at age 45. For more on screening recommendations, see Chapter 2.

Family history

Studies indicate that if your father or brother had prostate cancer, your risk of the disease is at least twice as great as that of the average American male. Depending on the number of relatives in your family with prostate cancer and the age at which they had it, your risk could be even higher. In families with a history of prostate cancer, the cancer generally occurs at a younger age.

Mutations or changes in genes such as BRCA1, BRCA2 and HOXB13, as well as Lynch Syndrome (hereditary non-polyposis colorectal cancer, or HNPCC) have been linked to increased risk of developing prostate cancer. These mutations cause problems with the body's ability to repair DNA errors or with normal gene function, increasing the risk of prostate cancer and other types of cancer. Breast cancer (both male and female), colorectal cancer, ovarian cancer, pancreatic cancer and melanoma may also occur in families with these inherited changes. (For more information on genetics and prostate cancer, see Chapter 6.)

Although age is the primary risk factor for BPH, family history also plays a role. Among men who experience BPH in their 40s or early 50s, many carry an inherited gene that predisposes them to the disease. However, just because you carry the gene doesn't mean the disease is inevitable — it simply increases your risk.

Controllable factors

The risk of prostate disease varies among different populations. Because these differences don't appear to be genetic, researchers suspect that environment and lifestyle factors also play a role in your risk of developing prostate problems. However, at the moment, there are more questions about what these factors might be than about how you can control them.

Environment

Researchers are studying whether exposure to certain substances at your job may play a role in increasing your cancer risk. Higher rates of prostate cancer can be found in certain professions, such as farmers, than can be found in men in other occupations. Exposure to certain pesticides used in farm work has been linked to an increased risk of aggressive prostate cancer.

Diet

There's some evidence that a diet high in saturated and trans fats may increase your risk of prostate cancer and of more advanced disease. The reason behind this isn't clear, though at least one study has hypothesized that high-fat diets may mimic the effects of cancer-causing genes.

Other studies suggest that diets high in total calories and high in calcium and dairy products may increase the risk of prostate cancer. More research is needed.

On a more positive note, there's evidence that suggests chemicals found in soy products and certain vegetables and fruits may lower your risk. Any dietary changes that can improve your overall health, such as limiting or avoiding red meat, may aid cancer prevention in general. (See Chapter 11 for additional dietary tips.)

Tobacco

Current research doesn't support that smoking increases your risk of developing prostate cancer. However, studies have found that smokers diagnosed with prostate cancer are at increased risk of dying from the disease. This finding needs to be confirmed by additional studies.

Supplemental hormones

Dehydroepiandrosterone (DHEA) is a hormone that occurs naturally in your body. It's thought to be a precursor hormone — a chemical that's easily converted into other hormones, such as testosterone and estrogen. While DHEA supplements have been touted as providing many benefits, none of those benefits has been proved in research. In fact, DHEA might increase the risk of hormone-sensitive cancers, including prostate, breast and ovarian cancers. If you have any form of cancer or are at risk of cancer, don't use DHEA.

Sexual activity

The impact of sexual activity on prostate cancer risk is controversial. Some past research suggested that men with a history of sexually transmitted infections (STIs) such as gonorrhea or chlamydia may be at higher risk of prostate cancer. However, a definitive relationship hasn't been proved and more research is needed. A recent study suggests that certain factors, such as fewer sexual partners over the course of a lifetime, may be associated with a lower prostate cancer risk.

ANSWERS TO YOUR QUESTIONS

Is it possible to be born with an abnormal prostate gland?

Yes. You can have a congenital abnormality in your prostate gland. Because of the prostate's location, men with congenital prostate abnormalities sometimes also have kidney abnormalities — affecting the function of both the urinary and reproductive systems. These conditions aren't common, however, and can easily be diagnosed with X-ray or ultrasound images of the prostate gland and the kidneys.

I once had a sexually transmitted disease. Does this increase my risk of having prostate problems?

It's possible, yes. Some sexually transmitted infections, such as gonorrhea and chlamydia, may cause inflammation of the urethra, the tube that carries urine out of your bladder. This inflammation can sometimes produce scar tissue that narrows or blocks the urethra, increasing your risk of infection of the lower urinary tract or infection in your prostate gland (prostatitis).

Is it true that a vasectomy can increase my risk of prostate cancer?

It's unclear if undergoing a vasectomy increases the risk of developing prostate cancer, with research producing inconsistent and contradictory findings. One large study that followed Danish men for almost 40 years found a statistically significant increased long-term risk of prostate cancer among men who had the procedure. One hypothesis is that testicular function may have protective benefits against prostate cancer, so a procedure such as a vasectomy that alters that function could have a negative impact. However, other studies have reported no increased risk. Overall, the evidence suggests that if there is any risk, it's very low.

Getting a prostate checkup

You are your own best protection against prostate disease. If you can help identify a prostate condition in its early stages, you have a better chance of successful treatment. How do you do that? By being aware of the signs and symptoms and by scheduling regular checkups with your doctor.

There's no set schedule for prostate checkups. Every man has a different makeup and medical history. If you're in your 40s or younger, an annual prostate screening generally isn't necessary unless you're experiencing prostate-related symptoms.

If you're between the ages of 40 and 54 and at a higher risk of prostate disease, discuss your situation with your doctor to determine if screening may be warranted.

Age is a major risk factor for prostate disease, and the older you are, the greater the likelihood of having problems with your prostate gland. Once you reach age 55, consider including an annual or biannual prostate examination as part of an overall physical checkup.

What's involved in a typical prostate exam varies, depending on your age, general health, medical history and lab test results from your previous checkup. Several tests may be performed, which are not conclusive by themselves but work well in combination.

Beyond a basic exam, other tests may be performed. These options may allow for a better estimation of your prostate disease risk, leading to earlier diagnosis and effective treatment.

SHARED DECISION-MAKING: CHOOSING THE RIGHT PATH FOR YOU

The decision to screen for prostate disease isn't always an easy one. A digital rectal exam (DRE) and prostate-specific antigen (PSA) test are often the first tools used to detect prostate cancer; however, these tests can lead to additional, more invasive testing and treatments with side effects that can significantly impact your quality of life. That's why a frank discussion with your doctor about the benefits and risks of screening is crucial.

Such discussions are part of a larger concept in health care called "shared decision-making." As the name implies, you and your doctor work together to reach the best course of care for you. Your doctor will discuss your risk factors — such as a family history of prostate disease, race and health history — and offer guidance based on these factors. Armed with this information, you decide if and when to begin screenings. For example, if you're a healthy 55-year-old with no symptoms of prostate disease, you may decide that you don't want to screen for prostate cancer just yet after discussing the pros and cons with your doctor. Your doctor will likely recommend revisiting the topic in a couple of years.

Though shared decision-making is individual, the goals are always the same: to get you and your doctor on the same page regarding your health care, avoid unnecessary treatments and side effects, and make sure you're comfortable with the medical care you receive.

BASIC TESTS

Many doctors include a prostate checkup as part of a male physical examination. In addition to standard procedures, such as checking your blood pressure and listening to your heart and lungs, your doctor may perform some or all of the following prostate-related exams or tests:
• Digital rectal examination.
• Urinalysis.
• PSA test.

Digital rectal examination

A digital rectal examination is a screening test for prostate disease, as well as for detecting other problems in the lower rectum. However, a digital rectal exam ranks among the least-desired parts of a physical exam because many men find it embarrassing or uncomfortable.

A digital rectal exam is, in fact, quick and painless. You'll be asked to bend forward

DIGITAL RECTAL EXAMINATION

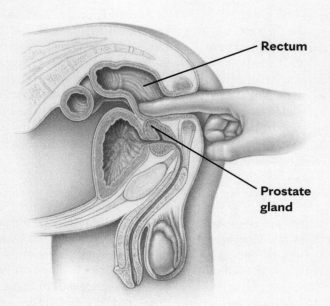

Rectum

Prostate gland

During a digital rectal examination, your doctor inserts a gloved, lubricated finger into your rectum and feels the back wall of the prostate gland for enlargement, tenderness, lumps or hard spots.

at the waist, with pants down, leaning against an exam table, or to lie on your side on the table with your knees pulled up to your chest.

After checking the outside of your anus for hemorrhoids or tiny breaks in the tissue (fissures), your doctor gently inserts a gloved finger, lubricated with gel, into your rectum.

Because the prostate gland is next to the rectum, your doctor can feel the back

wall of the prostate gland and examine the gland for bumps, irregularities, asymmetry, soft spots or hard spots in the prostate tissue that may suggest an abnormality.

A gland that feels enlarged may indicate benign prostatic hyperplasia (BPH). If the gland feels tender to the touch, it may be a sign of prostatitis. In addition, the outer portion of the gland is where 70% to 85% of cancerous tumors develop. In the early stages of development, prostate tumors often feel like nodules or hard spots.

A digital rectal exam doesn't provide conclusive results — rather, it's an indicator of whether additional tests are required. For example, just because your doctor may detect a hard spot on your prostate during the exam doesn't mean you have cancer. Other conditions, including prostate infection or the formation of small stones in the gland, can produce similar symptoms. Other tests are needed to help clarify the findings.

At the same time, just because abnormalities aren't identified doesn't mean there aren't any problems. A high percentage of prostate cancers, particularly in the early stages, are undetectable.

Although a digital rectal exam has long been used as a screening tool for prostate cancer, there's limited evidence of its effectiveness in decreasing prostate cancer deaths. Data from the long-term Prostate, Lung, Colorectal and Ovarian (PLCO) Cancer Screening Trial found no survival benefit after screening with a digital rectal exam and PSA test. Another study that found some benefit when screening with a PSA test noted that this benefit occurred regardless of being combined with a digital rectal exam.

Some past studies have shown prostate screening exams can be beneficial. One Mayo Clinic study found evidence that men who didn't receive regular digital rectal exams were more likely to die of prostate cancer than were a similar group of men who did have regular exams.

At this time, neither the American Urological Association nor the American Cancer Society gives definitive recommendations on digital rectal exams, while the U.S. Preventive Services Task Force does not recommend them. Mayo Clinic urologists recommend discussing the exam with your doctor if you're considering prostate screening.

Urine test

Urine is fluid that transports waste products out of your body. A urine test detects various compounds in urine that may indicate a problem. A urine sample is collected, checked for color and appearance, and analyzed under a microscope.

- If your urine contains more white blood cells than is normal, you may have an infection in your prostate gland (prostatitis) or urinary tract.
- Red blood cells in your urine may signal inflammation of the prostate or, perhaps, a tumor. Other conditions, including bladder problems or inflammation of the urethra, also can produce blood in your urine.
- A urine test that doesn't detect any abnormalities can help confirm a diagnosis of benign prostatic hyperplasia.

Prostate-specific antigen (PSA) test

PSA is a biological marker that can be used to detect disease. For this test, a blood sample is taken and analyzed for the antigen. PSA is a compound produced in your prostate gland that helps liquefy semen — an action essential to the reproductive process.

It's common for a small amount of PSA to circulate in your bloodstream. If higher-than-normal levels of PSA are measured in your blood, it could indicate prostate inflammation, enlargement or cancer.

Much as with a digital rectal exam, results from a PSA test aren't conclusive evidence that you have a prostate condition — some men with high PSA levels end up having no problems with their prostates. Rather, abnormal PSA test results indi-cate that you're at higher risk of disease and that more tests may be necessary to help clarify what's causing the increase.

A PSA test often is used in conjunction with a digital rectal exam for initial prostate screening. However, many questions remain regarding how to interpret PSA test results and whether these findings should guide the course of future evaluation and treatment.

THE PSA DEBATE

The PSA test was approved by the Food and Drug Administration in 1986 as a means to help detect prostate cancer.

MAYO CLINIC PSA STANDARDS

Mayo Clinic urologists use this age-adjusted scale in determining if PSA results are within standard limits for your age. The results are based on the test used at Mayo Clinic. The upper limit of what's considered normal increases as you age.

Age	Upper limit ng/mL*
<40	2.0
40-49	2.5
50-59	3.5
60-69	4.5
70-79	6.5
≥80	7.2

*Nanograms per milliliter

Since that time, including the test in standard physical exams has resulted in a significant increase in the recorded number of cases of prostate cancer. But controversy still remains concerning the dependability and utility of PSA test results.

The test begins with a small amount of blood drawn from your arm that's sent to a laboratory, where a specialized procedure called an immunochemical assay determines how much of the prostate-specific antigen is circulating in your bloodstream.

A reading between 0 and 4 nanograms per milliliter (ng/mL) is generally considered to be standard, or typical. However, because PSA levels tend to naturally increase as you get older, some medical centers have adjusted their standards based on age (see "Mayo Clinic PSA standards" on page 25).

Just because your PSA level is below the upper limit of normal doesn't rule out the presence of prostate cancer. Similarly, just because your PSA is elevated doesn't necessarily mean you have cancer. Some men have higher-than-normal PSA levels and healthy prostates.

It's also important to understand that other conditions or actions in addition to cancer can increase the amount of PSA in your bloodstream:
- **BPH.** Noncancerous enlargement of the prostate is the most common condition that can cause an elevated PSA reading. As prostate tissue grows, cells within the tissue produce more PSA — sometimes up to three times higher than is typical.
- **Prostatitis.** Irritation of the prostate gland due to inflammation or infection can cause cells to release or leak higher amounts of PSA into the bloodstream.
- **Urinary tract infection.** Similar to an infection in your prostate gland (prostatitis), a urinary tract infection can increase the PSA level in your blood.
- **Ejaculation.** The release of semen can cause a temporary increase in PSA levels. For that reason, some doctors have advised patients to abstain from sexual activity for up to 2 days before having their PSA exam.

In addition, procedures used to treat BPH (discussed in Chapter 5) can temporarily irritate the prostate gland, producing abnormal levels of PSA. These procedures include:
- Prostate biopsy.
- Transurethral resection of the prostate.
- Transurethral incision of the prostate.
- Microwave therapy of the prostate.
- Laser therapy of the prostate.

Following one of these procedures, you should wait 2 weeks to 2 months before having a PSA test.

Concerns

The PSA test is able to identify early-stage prostate cancer about 75% of the time. In about 25% of men with early-stage prostate cancer, PSA results come back within the standard range (less than 4 ng/mL). This is a major drawback of the test. If a PSA test is the only screening tool, early-stage prostate cancer in about 1 of 4 men will go undetected.

As mentioned earlier, another drawback of using PSA as a screening tool is that the results don't distinguish between cancer and other prostate diseases. Among men with elevated PSA levels who undergo a biopsy, 75% don't have cancer. Increased PSA levels in these men may be a result of BPH, prostatitis or other factors.

As a result, many men who don't have cancer undergo testing that's expensive, time-consuming and may be hard on their physical and emotional health.

Because of these drawbacks, not all doctors and medical organizations agree that the benefits of the PSA test outweigh its limitations. That's why this simple test remains controversial.

Benefits

The benefit of regular PSA screening is that it can help identify prostate cancer long before any signs or symptoms become apparent — often when the cancer is still confined to the prostate gland. Localized cancer is much easier to treat and cure than cancer that's spread to other organs and tissues in the body.

Not all prostate cancers are alike. Some cancers grow slowly and remain within the prostate gland. Others are more aggressive and spread rather quickly to other organs. If your PSA test detects what turns out to be an aggressive form of prostate cancer, it could be a lifesaver.

The year 1995 marked the first-ever reduction in deaths from prostate cancer. Many doctors believe, and some studies support, that the PSA test was a major factor behind this decrease. However, health experts haven't been able to prove this link with certainty.

Limitations

Among men for whom test results come back normal, the results may provide a false sense of security. And among men with an elevated PSA, the men may go through needless worry and unnecessary, expensive diagnostic procedures to learn they don't have cancer.

Whether the test leads to needless treatment is another question. If you have a slow-growing cancer, you may be able to monitor your condition and live with the cancer for years without it causing any problems.

Some men, however, find the waiting game difficult to accept. When they learn they have cancer, they want to do every-thing they can to get rid of it, opting for treatments such as surgery or radiation therapy. These treatments may lead to side effects, including incontinence or impotence. These conditions can de-crease the quality of life for men who might otherwise have enjoyed perfectly healthy, productive lives.

Finally, the issue of whether the early detection and treatment of prostate cancer actually saves lives remains unresolved. A large European study

BPH MEDICATIONS AND PSA

Finasteride (Proscar) and dutasteride (Avodart) are medications commonly used to treat BPH. They shrink the prostate gland by suppressing certain hormones that stimulate prostate growth. Finasteride is the same drug taken to promote hair growth in balding men, sold under the brand name Propecia.

By altering hormone levels in the prostate gland, these drugs reduce production of PSA in the gland. To compensate for this and get a more accurate reading, your doctor may double the PSA results. For example, if the standard range for a 70-year-old man is 0 to 6.5 ng/mL, and a man who is taking finasteride has a PSA level of 2.6 ng/mL, his true reading is 5.2, which puts him within the standard range.

It's essential for your doctor to be aware that you're taking these medications so that he or she can monitor and interpret your PSA results appropriately.

(European Randomized Study of Screening for Prostate Cancer, or ERSPC) comparing men who underwent PSA screening to those who didn't showed a significant reduction in prostate cancer deaths and risk for cancer spread (metastasis) among men who had PSA screening.

But another study conducted in the United States (Prostate, Lung, Colorectal and Ovarian Cancer Screening Trial, or PLCO) indicated there was no benefit in overall or cancer-specific survival with PSA screening. Specifically, trial data found that men who underwent annual prostate cancer screening (with PSA testing and a digital rectal exam) had a 12% higher incidence of prostate cancer than did men who didn't undergo routine screening exams. However, after 13 years of follow-up, researchers didn't find a

statistically significant difference in mortality rates between the two groups.

A caveat: While the control group in the PLCO trial didn't receive annual screening through the trial, the majority were screened at least once during the trial as part of their regular care. So, while the trial results found no survival benefit with annual screening as compared with opportunistic screening, there was no comparison of regular screening versus no screening as in the ERSPC trial.

CURRENT RECOMMENDATIONS

So, should you have a PSA test? There's still no definitive answer. There are a few organizations that recommend against PSA-based screenings. However, most organizations suggest discussing the risks and benefits of the test with your doctor in order to make an informed decision based on your risk factors and your values and preferences.

The American Cancer Society (ACS) recommends that men begin discussions with their doctors about prostate screening as follows:

- At age 40 for men at the highest risk. This includes men with more than one first-degree relative (father, brother or son) who developed prostate cancer before age 65.
- At age 45 for men at increased risk of developing prostate cancer. This includes Black men and men who have just one first-degree relative who was diagnosed with prostate cancer before age 65.
- At age 50 for men who are at average risk of prostate cancer and are expected to live at least 10 more years.

The American Urological Association (AUA) offers slightly different recommendations:

- For men under age 55, no routine screening. The exception is for men considered at higher risk (Black men or men with a family history of prostate cancer). Men at high risk should discuss prostate screening with their doctor according to their individual circumstances.
- For men between the ages of 55 and 69, a discussion with their doctors about the risks and benefits of prostate cancer screening. For men in this group, screening every 2 years may be preferred over annual screening, as this

may reduce overdiagnosis and false positives while still detecting cancer at the early stages.

The U.S. Preventive Services Task Force (USPSTF) takes an approach similar to the AUA:

- For men 55 to 69, the decision to undergo periodic PSA testing is individual and based on a discussion of the potential benefits and harms of screening, taking into account family history, race and ethnicity, other medical conditions and a person's preferences.

As for how long you should continue testing, the recommendations of most organizations are based on life expectancy. Some, like the USPSTF, suggest that screening not be offered to men older than age 70. However, the AUA notes that some men older than 70 who are in excellent health may still benefit from prostate cancer screening. Screening isn't typically recommended for men with a life expectancy of less than 10 to 15 years.

Mayo Clinic's view

Like the ACS, AUA and USPSTF, Mayo Clinic recommends an individualized approach to determining whether screening is appropriate for you. This involves taking into consideration your individual risk of developing prostate cancer, your overall health, and a discussion of the benefits and potential risks of screening.

Mayo Clinic recommends that men in their 50s and 60s with a life expectancy greater than 10 years discuss screening with their doctors. For men at increased risk — including Black men and men with a family history of prostate cancer — discussions regarding PSA screening should begin at age 40.

IMPROVING PSA TESTING

Researchers continue looking for a more accurate screening method that can reduce or eliminate some of the concerns regarding the current PSA test. New screening tools include blood, urine and tissue tests, which can help predict whether elevated PSA levels are related to cancer. And if cancer is present, certain tests may help better predict whether it's an aggressive or nonaggressive type. The goal is to identify which men may need additional testing or treatment.

Blood tests

PSA that circulates in your bloodstream comes in two forms — prostate-specific antigens bound to blood proteins and antigens that are unbound (free PSA). The PSA test most commonly used today measures both forms to determine the total amount of PSA in your blood.

Researchers have learned that getting separate readings of bound and unbound PSA — called a free-PSA test — may help determine the type of prostate disease you have. It turns out noncancerous conditions such as BPH are associated with higher levels of free PSA in blood, whereas prostate cancer is linked to higher levels of bound PSA. The lower the percentage of free PSA on your test results, the more likely the increase in PSA is associated with cancer. This would signal the need for more testing, including a prostate biopsy.

Other testing under evaluation includes the following tests:

PSA velocity

This is the rate of change in your PSA levels over time. The thought is that rapidly rising levels may signal prostate cancer. However, recent studies have cast doubt on the value of PSA velocity in identifying cancer. The American Cancer Society doesn't recommend using PSA velocity for prostate cancer screening.

Ultrasensitive PSA test

This specialized test is capable of detecting minute quantities of PSA in your bloodstream. If you've already been treated for prostate cancer, this test may detect a recurrence of cancer far earlier than other tests — perhaps by a year or two.

Prostate health index (PHI)

It takes the combined measurements of three types of PSA tests (PSA, free PSA and p2PSA). The p2PSA test measures a specific component (isoform) of free PSA. The resulting score predicts the probability of finding cancer on a prostate biopsy.

4Kscore

This blood test identifies four measurements — three types of PSA as well as the enzyme human kallikrein 2 (hK2) — and is used in a formula along with other risk-related information to calculate your risk of aggressive prostate cancer after an abnormal PSA or digital rectal exam.

PSA density test

The test compares your PSA level to the size of your prostate gland. What's known as prostate-specific antigen density (PSAD) is calculated by dividing your PSA level by your prostate volume. A higher PSAD generally indicates a greater likelihood of prostate cancer. To get an accurate prostate volume, you would need to undergo imaging of the prostate, using transrectal ultrasound or prostate MRI. Because it requires an additional procedure, use of PSA density remains problematic.

Urine tests

These tests look for specific genetic material in urine samples, which can indicate whether cancer or an aggressive form of cancer is present.

SelectMDx

The tests look for two genes (DLX1 and HOXC6) in a urine sample obtained after a digital rectal exam. The testing is designed to help identify patients with clinically significant prostate cancer who would benefit from a prostate biopsy.

ExoDX

This test looks for three biomarkers associated with aggressive prostate cancer — ERG, PCA and SPDEF. It doesn't analyze PSA. A prostate exam isn't needed before this test.

PCA3

Among men with prostate cancer, the prostate cancer gene 3 is highly overexpressed. This overexpression is detectable with a urine test done after a prostate exam. A PCA3 score gives the likelihood of a positive biopsy.

MiPs

The test looks for the presence of genetic materials from the PCA3 gene and T2-ERG, which results from the fusion of two different genes. Both are strong indicators of prostate cancer.

Tissue tests

Tissue testing examines noncancerous prostate tissue taken during a biopsy to help determine which men may need follow-up testing or procedures. The ConfirmMDx test is a molecular test that looks at three biomarkers (GSTP1, RASSF1, APC) associated with prostate cancer. The test is typically used in men who have elevated or increasing PSA levels or an abnormal digital rectal exam and negative results on a previous biopsy to determine if a repeat biopsy may be needed.

ANSWERS TO YOUR QUESTIONS

Can my family doctor do a prostate examination?

Absolutely. Family physicians are vital to the process of screening men for prostate cancer or other abnormalities. A digital rectal exam and PSA testing are routine, and virtually every family doctor is familiar with them. You and your doctor can work together to come up with an examination and testing schedule that you're comfortable with. (See the section "Shared decision-making" on page 22.)

When should I see a urologist?

Your family doctor may recommend that you see a urologist if he or she has questions regarding your test results, suspects prostate cancer or believes a urologist could better treat noncancerous conditions such as BPH or prostatitis. If you have a problem urinating, your PSA level is elevated, or your family doctor finds an abnormality during a digital rectal exam, you may want to see a urologist.

My PSA level has always been very low. It's still within the normal range, but it has increased. Should I be concerned?

As you age, your PSA level may increase slightly. However, a noticeable change in your PSA should be followed up with a thorough evaluation, even if the reading is within the normal range.

Imaging procedures

Seeing inside the body is often necessary for a doctor to correctly diagnose and treat a prostate condition. Today, sophisticated imaging technology permits a doctor to study the structure and function of internal organs and identify abnormal conditions without the risk and discomfort of exploratory surgery.

Often, imaging techniques are used in conjunction with various treatment options to minimize the negative side effects of treatment while obtaining the best possible results.

In discussions with your doctor about a prostate problem, you'll undoubtedly hear references to imaging procedures such as ultrasound, computerized tomography (CT) and magnetic resonance imaging (MRI). What do the different images show? How will the procedures help you? Are there any health risks or side effects to be aware of?

This section may answer some of your questions and alleviate some of your concerns. The following pages describe specific techniques used for diagnosing prostate concerns and show the images these techniques produce.

This information may help you better understand their importance in your health care and the role of the procedures in making treatment decisions.

The type of imaging recommended for you will depend on the symptoms you are experiencing and the results of screening tests such as a digital rectal exam and PSA test.

Cystoscopy

A cystoscope is a thin tube that can be inserted into your urethra and bladder. The tube is equipped with a small camera and light to display visuals on an external monitor — allowing your doctor to guide the device and see inside the structures. The scope can be manipulated in different directions by your doctor.

The scope also contains open channels through which tiny instruments can be inserted to perform minor procedures, eliminating the need for incisions or open surgery — for example, removing tissue samples from the prostate or bladder (biopsy).

Cystoscopy is used to diagnose problems of the urinary tract and prostate, including polyps, tumors and unusual growths, cancer, infection or inflammation, and causes of obstructed or painful urination.

When this device is used in other parts of the body, the procedure is called endoscopy. Cystoscopy is specific to an examination of the urinary tract.

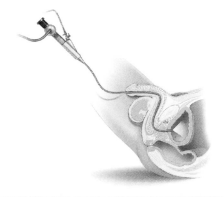

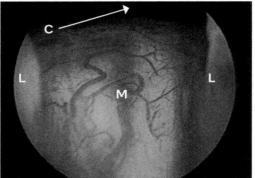

A cystographic image of the urethra at the apex of the prostate (arrow A). The ejaculatory duct is visible (arrow B), connecting the prostate and seminal vesicles for the production of sperm.

A cystographic image of the urethra at the bladder neck (arrow C). Two lateral lobes (L) and median lobe (M) of the prostate are visible.

Ultrasound

For an ultrasound procedure, a technician gently presses a small device (transducer) against your skin that emits high-frequency sound waves. Tissues and fluids inside your body, all of varying densities, reflect the sound waves back to the transducer. This device collects the echoes and relays them to a computer, which generates the image. The strength of an echo depends on the density of the tissue it's reflected from and how far away the tissue is.

Ultrasound images capture the function and movement of internal organs in real time, such as the narrowing of vessels and blockage of blood flow. Ultrasound can also guide doctors through delicate procedures such as a needle biopsy or focused ablation.

In a transrectal ultrasound, the transducer is attached to a probe and inserted into your rectum to get a better view of your prostate gland. The image can determine whether your prostate is enlarged but is not as effective in detecting abnormal growths or suspicious areas within the organ.

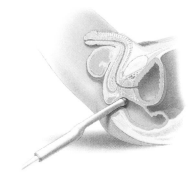

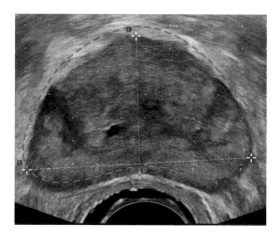

This transrectal ultrasound view shows a healthy prostate (red outline). The rectum (red arrow) is located behind the prostate.

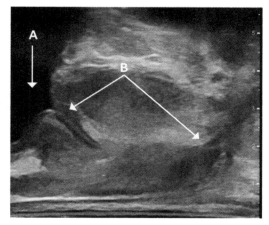

This ultrasound view shows a healthy prostate with the bladder (arrow A) and urethra (B arrows).

X-ray

An X-ray machine emits a small burst of electromagnetic radiation through your body, which passes through bones, organs and soft tissue. Special film positioned behind the part of your body being X-rayed collects the signal, generating a 2D image of your internal structures.

Different kinds of tissue absorb different amounts of the radiation. Dense tissue such as bone absorbs radiation well, so a weak signal reaches the film — bone appears as white on the film. Muscle and fat allow more radiation to pass through than bone does, so they appear on X-ray film in different shades of gray. Hollow structures, such as the intestines, absorb little radiation, and they appear dark on the film.

Sometimes, contrast dye will be added into your system to make hollow or fluid-filled structures such as the bladder or a blood vessel more visible on an X-ray. In this way, X-rays can also indicate the location of a polyp, tumor or obstruction.

A test that uses X-ray imaging and a contrast dye to look at the urinary system is called an excretory urogram. This test has been replaced in most cases by a CT urogram. In case of a blockage in the urethra, contrast dye also can be inserted into the urethra via a catheter to outline an area and help identify the problem.

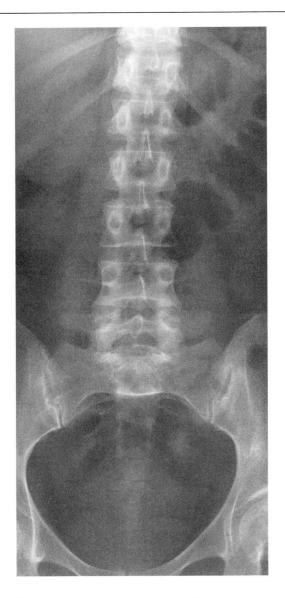

The image above is a standard X-ray of the abdomen and pelvic region. Dense tissue such as bone is the most prominently visible feature.

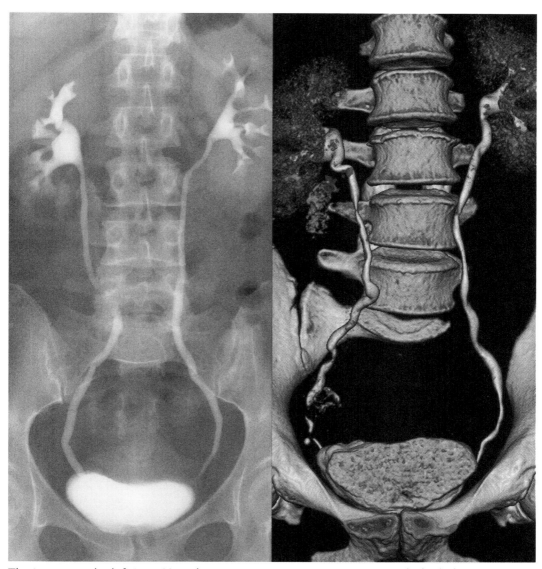

The image on the left is an X-ray known as an excretory urogram. With the help of contrast dye, a series of images taken at regular intervals reveals the kidneys, ureters and bladder — organs that may not show up well on a standard X-ray. In the image on the right, special software has compiled the information into a volume-rendered, 3D picture.

Computerized tomography (CT)

CT combines X-rays with computers. The procedure makes multiple scans of your internal organs and tissue. Think of a loaf of bread that's been cut into slices — each CT image represents a thin, cross-sectional slice of your body.

Standard X-rays are created by a stationary machine that focuses radiation on one part of your body. CT scans involve a sophisticated X-ray unit that rotates around your body, emitting a series of radiation beams. An X-ray detector rotates opposite this source, on the other side of your body, collecting the signals.

This procedure can detect hundreds of different levels of tissue density, in contrast to standard X-rays, which detect only a few levels of density. A CT scan has a much greater degree of detail and clarity than standard X-rays.

For the procedure, you lie on a table (gantry) that slides through a ring-shaped structure containing the X-ray unit. Small doses of radiation pass through your body at slightly different angles as the gantry slowly moves through the ring. A computer gathers the radiation signals. Each signal is interpreted on a scale ranging from black to white, according to the signal's intensity.

A CT scan can locate stones, tumors, infections, obstructions and cancer. Doctors also use this form of imaging to guide procedures such as biopsies and surgeries.

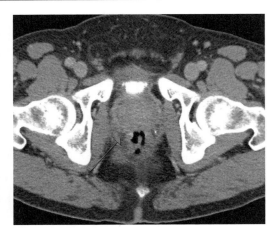

This CT image shows a healthy prostate (red arrow) and the pelvic region, taken in the axial plane. The hip bones are the large, white structures.

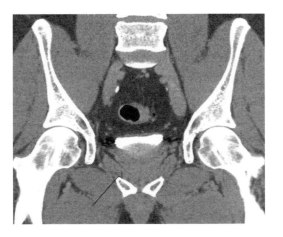

This CT image shows a healthy prostate (red arrow) and pelvic region taken in the coronal plane.

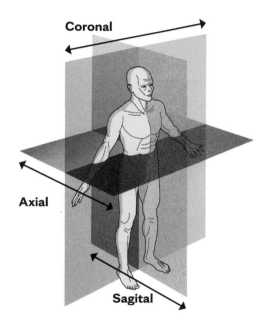

Coronal

Axial

Sagital

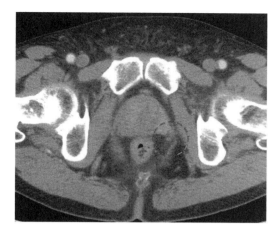

This axial CT image indicates the presence of cancer that has spread beyond the prostate — known as extraprostatic extension (red circle).

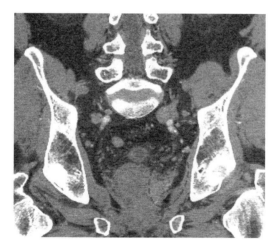

This CT image provides a coronal view of the same extraprostatic extension that's pictured in the axial CT image above (red oval).

Magnetic resonance imaging (MRI)

MRI creates cross-sectional pictures of internal organs, soft tissues and other structures, which can assist a doctor in diagnosing and treating prostate problems. MRI differs from CT because it uses a magnetic field and radio waves instead of radiation to create images. MRI scans provide much greater detail and clarity of soft tissues than do CT scans, especially of the prostate gland.

Typically, an MRI machine consists of a long, cylindrical scanner equipped with strong magnets. The magnetic field aligns some of the atomic particles in your body.

The aligned particles are influenced by complex radiofrequency pulses to produce tiny signals that can be detected by a computer and made into images.

MRI can be used to diagnose, treat and monitor a variety of conditions, including abnormalities of the urinary or reproductive tracts, infection or enlargement of the prostate gland, and cancer, including prostate and bladder cancers. MRI may also be used to guide targeted diagnostic procedures, such as a biopsy, and to guide and monitor prostate cancer therapies such as ablation.

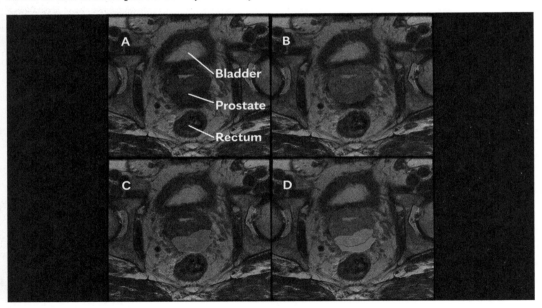

MRI image A shows the bladder, prostate gland and rectum; image B identifies the borders (capsule) of the prostate gland (shaded green); image C indicates cancer (shaded yellow) within the prostate; image D indicates cancer that has spread outside the prostate capsule (shaded red).

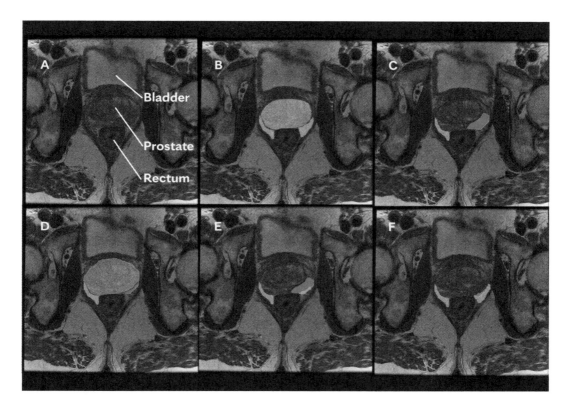

MRI image A shows the bladder, prostate gland and rectum; image B identifies the borders (capsule) of the prostate gland (shaded blue) and the nerve bundles on both sides of the gland (shaded teal); images C and D show cancer in the prostate gland in close proximity to a nerve bundle (shaded red); image E depicts spread of the cancer into the adjacent nerve bundle (shaded orange); image F depicts how much of the bundle has been invaded by cancer (shaded red).

MRI-ultrasound fusion

Advances in MRI technology involve a combination of features that are displayed in separate, unique imaging sequences during an MRI exam. This allows for better detection and characterization of masses within the prostate gland.

Some of the imaging sequences require specialized software for analysis and interpretation, as shown below.

Digital imaging systems make it possible for a doctor to rapidly analyze multiple image views that are created during a prostate MRI. The ability to see multiple images at the same time can provide a clearer diagnosis and help to determine a course of treatment. Additional technology may then be used to guide treatment in real time.

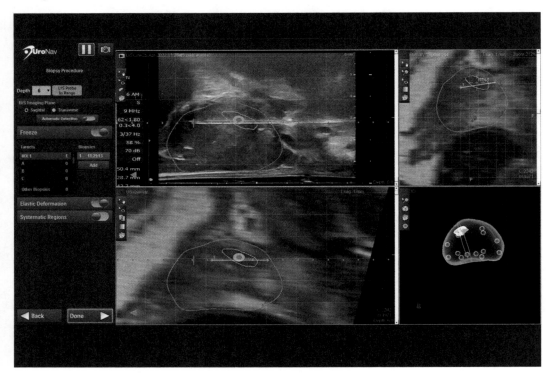

These images show a prostate gland with a noted tumor. The details are rather complex, but they demonstrate how specialized MRI-fusion software allows doctors to analyze images and data in a synchronized, clear way. The technology makes it possible to target and guide optimal placement of a biopsy needle.

Nuclear scan

Nuclear scanning — a subspecialty of radiology — introduces tiny amounts of radioactive materials called tracers (radionuclides) into your body to help visualize and evaluate medical conditions. The tracers travel through your bloodstream and accumulate in certain designated tissues.

Wherever their location in your body, the tracers emit gamma radiation, which is detected by a special camera that can generate images of the internal structures as well as the biochemical processes taking place.

Different radionuclides are designed to go to different organs and tissues, so the tracer selected for your test will depend on your symptoms. For example, one type of tracer collects in bone, while another goes to the kidneys. How much tracer is absorbed into the tissue may indicate the type of problem and how serious it is.

Nuclear scans provide different information than do an X-ray and ultrasound images. The information is based on biological changes rather than structural ones. A radioactive tracer can sometimes detect disease at earlier stages than other diagnostic tests can — a critical factor in effectively treating prostate cancer.

Nuclear scans can be superimposed over other imaging to correlate information from the different procedures. This process is known as image fusion.

Different kinds of nuclear imaging tests include bone scans, renal scans and positron emission tomography (PET). All of the procedures are important in diagnosing and treating prostate disease. Some are discussed in upcoming pages.

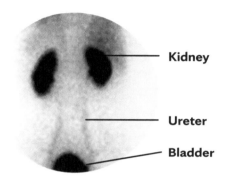

A renal scan showing the kidneys and bladder.

Bone scan

A bone scan is a form of nuclear imaging in which tracers (radioactive materials) injected into your body accumulate in your bones. Radiation emitted by these tracers is detected by a special camera. The scan reveals the metabolic state of your bones — the natural processes of bone growth, decay and renewal.

Specialists will study the scan looking for evidence of abnormal metabolism. Tracer material that accumulates in healthy bone shows up in medium tones. Darker "hot spots" and lighter "cold spots" indicate where the tracer has or hasn't accumulated — often an indication of a problem.

Changes in metabolism can result from various problems, including tumors and joint infections. More importantly, a scan can reveal the presence of cancer, which may have spread (metastasized) from another location (red ovals).

Healthy

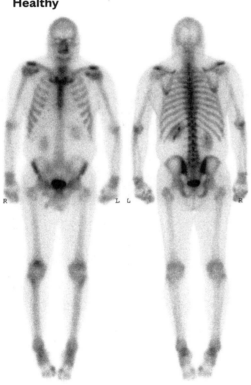

Metastasis

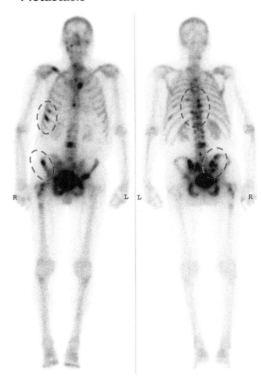

Positron emission tomography (PET)

PET is a form of nuclear imaging that measures the chemical processes taking place in your body. The test can help doctors distinguish between normal and abnormal functions of different organs and tissues.

For a PET scan, you receive an injection of a radioactive drug called a tracer. A short time later, a special scanner is used to detect where the tracer collects in your body. Cells that take up the majority of the drug appear on the scan as bright, intense colors, or "hot spots." Cells that don't take up as much of the drug appear as less intense colors, or "cold spots."

For example, cancerous tissue often will take up more tracer and appear as a hot spot on a PET scan. This helps your doctor determine spread of the cancer (metastasis) or assess how the cancer is responding to treatment.

However, a PET scan must be interpreted carefully, and a biopsy is usually required to confirm the presence of cancer.

Historically, PET scans were reserved for men whose prostate cancer may have spread after treatment — for example, men who completed surgery or radiation therapy but are now faced with rising PSA levels and suspected metastasis.

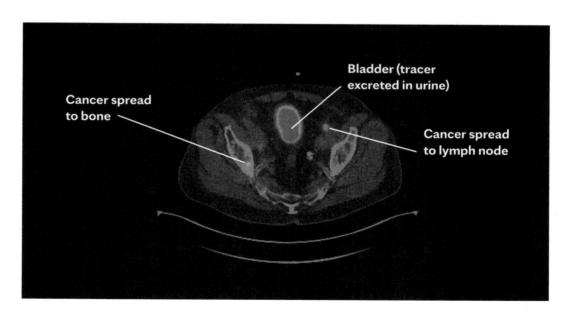

This PET image reveals cancer that has spread outside the prostate gland (metastatic cancer).

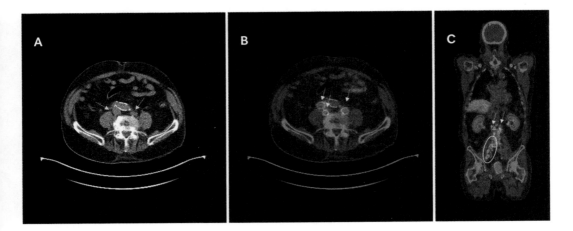

Image A shows questionable lymph node involvement in the uppermost pelvic region (yellow arrows); image B reveals increased activity in these lymph nodes, suggesting metastatic cancer (yellow arrows); image C reveals increased activity in multiple lymph nodes in the upper pelvis and peritoneal region, suggestive of high-volume prostate cancer (yellow arrows and circled area).

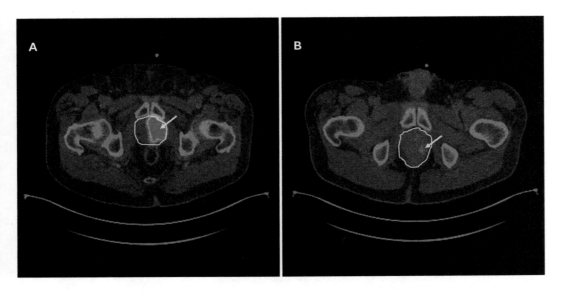

The images here show cancer that's confined to the prostate gland (localized cancer). Image A reveals a high level of activity in one half of the prostate gland (yellow arrow). Image B shows mild PSMA activity indicative of a low-grade cancer (yellow arrow).

Today, prostate-specific membrane antigen (PSMA) tracers are also approved for use at initial diagnosis when doctors suspect the cancer may not be confined to the prostate gland. There are several types of PET scan tracers approved for use in the diagnosis of prostate cancer. They include gallium-68 PSMA-11, piflufolastat F 18 PSMA, choline C-11, fluciclovine F 18 and sodium fluoride F 18.

PET scans are often fused with other imaging, such as CT or MRI. In fact, many PET scanners are equipped with CT or MRI technology.

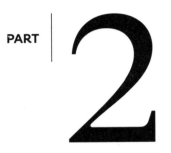

Noncancerous conditions

3

Prostatitis and chronic pelvic pain

One of the most common prostate problems men encounter in their lifetimes is one you seldom hear about — unless you're a doctor. According to some estimates, up to a quarter of all visits men make to a doctor for genital or urinary problems are related to prostatitis and pain in the pelvic region.

Prostatitis is a general term for inflammation of the prostate gland. Pelvic pain describes pain that primarily occurs between the scrotum and anus — an area referred to as the perineum. Pelvic pain may be a symptom of another condition, or it can be a condition in its own right.

If the pain lasts six months or longer, it's classified as chronic. There are many possible causes of chronic pelvic pain, including various disorders of the gastro-intestinal, urinary or reproductive systems, as well as disruption of the muscles or nerves. Diagnosing pelvic pain involves a process of elimination until the most likely cause can be determined.

Chronic pelvic pain can frequently develop in men; most commonly, it occurs in the form of prostatitis. Sometimes the symptoms are a result of persistent inflammation of the prostate gland. Other times, the pain isn't related to the prostate at all and is potentially related to issues with other structures throughout the pelvic region.

This chapter examines different types of prostatitis, as well as frequent triggers of chronic pelvic pain. You'll also learn about effective ways to manage both of these common concerns.

TYPES OF PROSTATITIS

Prostatitis is poorly understood and difficult to diagnose. In fact, many cases diagnosed as prostatitis end up involving the entire pelvic region.

Inflammation of the prostate gland may be due to an infection or another factor that's irritating the gland. The condition isn't contagious and it's not a sexually transmitted infection.

The National Institutes of Health (NIH) has classified four distinct types (categories) of prostatitis:
* Category I: acute bacterial prostatitis.
* Category II: chronic bacterial prostatitis.
* Category III: chronic pelvic pain syndrome (chronic prostatitis), including the conditions previously known as nonbacterial prostatitis and prostatodynia.
* Category IV: asymptomatic inflammatory prostatitis.

The first three types of prostatitis cause a variety of symptoms, including a frequent and urgent need to urinate and painful or burning sensations while urinating. This is often accompanied by pelvic, groin or low back pain. The fourth type has no symptoms. Identifying which type you have is crucial for successfully treating the condition.

Unlike other prostate problems, you're more likely to develop prostatitis when you're younger — even younger than age 40. You're also at increased risk if you:
* Recently had an infection of the bladder or urethra.

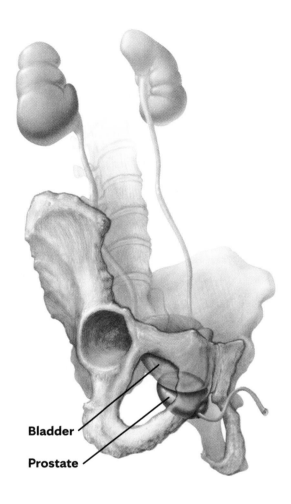

Bladder

Prostate

The urinary system and your prostate. The prostate gland is tucked into the pelvic region just below the bladder. Inflammation of the prostate may cause many urinary problems, as well as fever, chills and flu-like symptoms.

- Recently had a catheter inserted into your urethra.
- Don't empty your bladder frequently enough and perform vigorous activities with a full bladder.
- Jog or bicycle on a regular basis or ride horses.

Men with HIV also are at increased risk of developing one of the bacterial forms of prostatitis.

Pain relievers and several weeks of antibiotic treatment are typically needed to treat categories I and II prostatitis. Additional therapy, as well as self-care measures, also may provide relief. Treatment for category III prostatitis is less certain and directed toward relieving symptoms. Category IV prostatitis often doesn't require treatment.

Acute bacterial prostatitis

This form of prostatitis is the least common but most evident form of the disease. A bacterial infection in the prostate gland produces a sudden, severe onset of signs and symptoms. These may include a combination of:
- Fever and chills.
- Flu-like symptoms.
- Pain in the lower back, genital area or perineum.
- Urinary problems, including increased urgency and frequency, difficulty or pain when urinating, inability to completely empty the bladder, and blood-tinged urine.
- Sexual problems, including painful ejaculation and erectile dysfunction.

Bacteria normally found in the urinary tract or large intestine are most often responsible for this form of prostatitis. Most often, an acute infection starts in the prostate gland, but it can also spread from the bladder or urethra.

Acute bacterial prostatitis can lead to serious problems, including an inability to urinate and infection in the bloodstream (bacteremia). It's important to see your doctor immediately. Severe symptoms may require hospitalization for a few days until they improve.

Chronic bacterial prostatitis

Category II prostatitis also is caused by a bacterial infection. Typically, signs and symptoms develop gradually and they're often less severe than the acute form. They may include:
- Urinary problems, including increased urgency and frequency, difficulty starting or continuing urination, and diminished urine flow.
- Pain or burning sensation when urinating.
- Excessive nighttime urination.
- Pain in the lower back and genital area.
- Occasional blood in the semen (hematospermia).
- Sexual problems, including painful ejaculation and erectile dysfunction.
- Slight fever.
- Recurring bladder infection.

What causes the chronic infection often isn't clear. Sometimes chronic disease develops after an episode of acute prostatitis, when bacteria remain in the prostate. Other causes may include a bladder or blood infection or trauma to your urinary tract that may occur from activities such as bicycling or horseback riding.

Insertion of an instrument or catheter into your urethra, which may carry bacteria with it, is another potential cause of chronic infection. That's why some doctors prescribe antibiotics after use of a urinary catheter. Sometimes, stones form within prostate tissue, serving as a location for recurring infection. On rare occasions, prostatitis may result from an underlying structural or anatomical defect, which becomes a collection site for bacteria.

This form of prostatitis becomes chronic because the infection has penetrated deep into prostate tissue. Even if antibiotics reach the bacteria, the infection may persist and cause symptoms.

Chronic pelvic pain syndrome

Most men with prostatitis have the category III form. Unfortunately, this form is also the most difficult to diagnose and treat. Instead of trying to eliminate the disease, the primary goals of treatment are often to relieve symptoms and improve quality of life.

When the National Institutes of Health revised its classification system for prostatitis, it merged several conditions into category III that had previously been considered separate conditions, including chronic nonbacterial prostatitis and prostatodynia. This change was a recognition that symptoms often involve more than just the prostate gland.

Chronic pelvic pain is a syndrome — a collection of signs and symptoms that occur in a recognizable sequence or pattern. In diagnosing the condition, a

---

WHAT IS PROSTATODYNIA?

Prostatodynia is a category III form of prostatitis. Men who have prostatodynia often describe the condition as a dull pain "down there," meaning anywhere in the genital area. However, rather than being a problem with the prostate gland, prostatodynia may instead stem from the pelvic floor muscles.

When you're under stress, you may not completely relax the muscles supporting your bladder and urethra, causing difficulties when you urinate. This theory could explain why most men with these symptoms tend to have Type A personalities — hard-driven, tense and stressed. Prostatodynia also seems to occur frequently among marathon runners, bicyclists, triathletes, weightlifters and truck drivers.

doctor needs to evaluate many factors, including the location of pain and discomfort, severity of the symptoms, problems with urination, and impact on quality of life. In fact, the signs and symptoms of chronic pelvic pain syndrome are very similar to those for chronic bacterial prostatitis — both in kind and severity — although it's unlikely that you'll develop a fever.

This form of the disease is generally distinguished from a bacterial form of prostatitis with lab tests to determine whether bacteria are present in urine or prostate gland fluid. With chronic pelvic pain syndrome, lab tests don't find bacteria in the samples but on occasion may detect white blood cells — a sign of inflammation within the prostate.

The main reason why this form of prostatitis is difficult to treat is because the cause is uncertain. Theories abound as to possible triggers. However, no factors are definite, and many aren't well understood. Among the possible causes are:

- **Heavy lifting.** Lifting heavy objects while your bladder is full may cause urine to back up and seep into your prostate, causing inflammation.
- **Sexual activity.** Sexually active young men who have an inflammation of the urethra (urethritis) or sexually transmitted infection, such as gonorrhea or chlamydia, are more likely to develop the syndrome. In some men, having less sexual intercourse also may be a contributing factor.
- **Anxiety or stress.** They may cause you to tighten the urinary sphincter muscle — which controls urine flow from the bladder — and the muscles supporting your bladder and rectum (pelvic floor muscles). This prevents the muscles from relaxing, which may irritate your prostate or cause fluids in the urethra to back up into the prostate.
- **Pelvic muscle spasm.** Urinating in an uncoordinated manner when the internal sphincter muscle isn't relaxed may lead to increased pressure and inflammation in the prostate gland.
- **Other infectious agents.** The inflammation may be associated with a nonbacterial infectious agent that standard laboratory tests haven't detected.
- **Occupational factors.** Certain occupations, such as truck driving or operating heavy machinery, subject the prostate to a great deal of vibration.
- **Physical activities.** Activities such as bicycling or jogging may irritate the prostate gland if done frequently.

Whatever the initial trigger, the combination of inflammation and nerve irritation can result in chronic nerve sensitization — a process in which pain messages being sent to the brain are overly severe and out of proportion to the circumstances.

Sensitization may affect entire neurological pathways, including the sensing, feeling and thinking centers of your brain. Once nerve activation of this kind is established, many factors can stimulate the sensitized pathways and cause frequent symptom flares — for example, excessive amounts of caffeine or high levels of stress may bring on the condition.

Asymptomatic inflammatory prostatitis

Inflammation can occur in the prostate without producing any symptoms, which is why the name for this category IV form of prostatitis includes the word asymptomatic. Typically, the condition is discovered indirectly — for example, during a biopsy to check prostate tissue for cancer.

The cause of asymptomatic inflammation in the prostate is unknown. In addition, little is known about its long-term effects, and there are no effective means of treating it. While asymptomatic inflammatory prostatitis isn't cancerous, there's some speculation that it could be a precursor to prostate cancer. More research is needed to understand this condition.

DIAGNOSING PROSTATITIS

Most men have a prostate checkup in conjunction with their regular physical exams. If your doctor doesn't perform a digital rectal exam when you have a routine physical, ask whether you should have one.

It's also important to see your doctor if you develop any of the signs and symptoms of prostatitis, such as persistent urinary discomfort and pain, blood-tinged urine or semen, or pain while ejaculating — especially if these symptoms come on suddenly.

When left untreated, prostatitis can lead to more serious problems; for example, the infection could spread to other parts of your body.

Two important steps in diagnosing prostatitis are ruling out any other condition that may be causing the symptoms and determining the type of prostatitis you have. To start, you'll likely be asked questions about your symptoms: What are they? Do they come and go, or are they persistent? When did they first occur? Can you recall any changes in your lifestyle that took place about the time the symptoms began?

You also may be asked about recent medical procedures you've had, previous infections, your sexual habits, your occupation, and whether you have a family history of prostate problems. Often, a urine sample is collected at the beginning of the exam to check for evidence of a urinary tract infection.

A physical examination for prostatitis generally includes checking your abdomen and pelvic area for unusual tenderness. During a digital rectal exam, your doctor manually examines your prostate gland by gently inserting a lubricated, gloved finger into your rectum (see page 23). An inflamed prostate often feels enlarged and tender to the touch.

Prostate fluid also may be collected for evaluation during a rectal exam. Your doctor will rub vigorously against your prostate gland with a gloved finger, forcing the fluid into your urethra, where it combines with urine and exits through the penis. This procedure is often referred to as prostate massage or prostate stripping. A urine sample is then taken that includes fluid from the prostate massage. This fluid is examined under a microscope for evidence of bacteria and white blood cells. The presence of bacteria points to an infection. White blood cells indicate inflammation.

If your urine tests positive for both inflammation and infection, you likely have bacterial prostatitis, which can be treated with antibiotics. If the sample includes white blood cells but no bacteria, you probably have a form of chronic pelvic pain syndrome, in which the goal is symptom relief. If neither bacteria nor white blood cells are found in the urine sample, your symptoms may be related to other disorders.

If a cause isn't clear and to make sure your symptoms aren't related to other prostate conditions, such as cancer or benign prostatic hyperplasia (BPH), a doctor may order additional tests. They may include a prostate-specific antigen (PSA) test and tests to measure urine flow rate and residual volume after urination.

For some men, a doctor may recommend evaluation with X-rays, ultrasound, cystoscopy and specialized studies of bladder function. These tests may reveal tumors, bladder or urethral dysfunction, and other kidney or bladder problems.

TREATING PROSTATITIS

Once the category of prostatitis you have has been determined, you and your doctor can work together to develop a plan to treat the condition and, for the bacterial forms, possibly cure it.

Since the cause of chronic pelvic pain syndrome (category III) is often unknown, treating it is difficult. However, with some patience and experimentation, many men find ways to manage the condition and keep it from interfering with their daily lives. For many men, a combination of approaches is the most effective at controlling symptoms.

Medications

One or more of the following drugs may help eliminate or control your symptoms. Often, the medications are most effective early in the course of the treatment and become less effective over time.

Antibiotics

Antibiotics are generally the first line of treatment for all forms of prostatitis. Your doctor will likely start you on an antibiotic that fights a broad spectrum of bacteria. If the specific type of bacterium that's causing your infection can be identified based on urine and prostate fluid samples, a different drug may be prescribed that's more effective at killing that particular bacterium.

How long you'll take an antibiotic depends on how well you respond to the medication. For acute bacterial prostatitis, you may need medication for a few weeks, and you may need to be hospitalized and receive the antibiotics intravenously.

Chronic bacterial prostatitis is often more resistant to antibiotics, making the medications less effective. It takes longer to cure the infection — often 6 to 12 weeks — and sometimes it may never be eliminated. In addition, you may have a relapse as soon as you stop taking the antibiotic. To keep the infection under control, you may need to take a daily low-dose antibiotic for an indefinite period.

Even though chronic pelvic pain syndrome isn't associated with a bacterial infection, some doctors will prescribe an antibiotic for a few weeks to see if it improves symptoms. For unknown reasons, some men seem to benefit from a continuous low dose of an antibiotic.

Alpha blockers

If you're having difficulty urinating, perhaps due to an obstruction in your urinary tract, your doctor may prescribe an alpha blocker. Alpha blockers help relax the bladder neck and muscle fibers where the prostate gland adjoins the bladder. This can improve urine flow and help empty your bladder more completely.

Alpha blockers may also decrease the backflow of urine into the prostate, which may help control prostatitis. Side effects of alpha blockers can include reduced or absent ejaculation.

5-alpha reductase inhibitors

This class of drugs interferes with the effect of male hormones (androgens) on the prostate gland, which cause the prostate to enlarge. The medication stops the growth of the prostate gland and may even reduce its size. This may help relieve pain or urination problems caused by prostatitis.

A past study found that long-term use of the 5-alpha reductase inhibitor medication dutasteride (Avodart) caused an improvement in prostate symptoms among men ages 50 to 75 when compared with men who received an inactive substance (placebo). Studies involving the 5-alpha reductase inhibitor medication finasteride (Proscar) have produced mixed results.

While 5-alpha reductase inhibitors are common treatments for older men with urinary symptoms, they may not be recommended for men in their child-bearing years because of their effects on semen volume.

Pain relievers

Over-the-counter pain relievers, such as aspirin, ibuprofen (Advil, Motrin IB, others) and acetaminophen (Tylenol, others), can help relieve pain and discomfort. They may also help break the pain cycle brought on by sensitized nerves.

Keep in mind that taking too much of any of these medications can cause serious side effects, including abdominal pain and intestinal bleeding. Check first with your doctor before taking any pain reliever.

LIFESTYLE CHANGES

For reasons that are unclear, some men with chronic prostatitis find that making simple lifestyle changes, such as avoiding long periods of sitting or not eating certain foods and beverages, seems to improve their condition. Some of the more common practices include:

- Drinking plenty of water.
- Limiting alcohol, caffeine and highly spiced foods.
- Going to the bathroom at regular intervals.
- Having regular sexual activity.
- Using a "split" bicycle seat that reduces pressure on the prostate (if you're a bicyclist).

Although these practices don't appear to cause any harm, studies have yet to show that changes in dietary, bathroom or sexual habits can cure prostatitis or relieve its symptoms. If you find such practices helpful, continue them. Living with chronic prostatitis often comes down to limiting some things that seem to make the condition worse and doing other things that seem to improve it — without knowing why or how the changes help.

It's OK to experiment with various lifestyle changes, but do so gradually and always inform your doctor what you're doing.

Muscle relaxants

Pelvic muscle spasms may accompany prostatitis. On rare occasions, combining muscle relaxants with other medications to treat prostatitis may be helpful.

Other drugs

Other medications that may be considered include pregabalin (Lyrica), an anticonvulsant drug that's used to relieve pain from damaged nerves, and pentosan polysulfate sodium (Elmiron), a medication approved to treat interstitial cystitis, also known as painful bladder syndrome. Other medications, including corticosteroids and tricyclic antidepressants, are under investigation.

Physical therapy

Special exercises and relaxation techniques can improve symptoms in some men, perhaps because tight or irritated muscles may be contributing to the condition. Common techniques include the following.

PROSTATITIS SYMPTOM INDEX

Record answers to the following questions that best describe your symptoms. Discuss your answers with your doctor.

Pain or discomfort

1. In the last week, have you had any pain or discomfort in the following areas?
    a. Area between the rectum and the testicles (perineum).
    b. Testicles.
    c. Tip of the penis (not related to urination).
    d. Below the waist, in the pubic or bladder area.

2. In the last week, have you experienced:
    a. Pain or burning during urination?
    b. Pain or discomfort during or after sexual climax?

3. How often have you had pain or discomfort in any of these areas over the last week?
    0. Never   1. Rarely   2. Sometimes   3. Often   4. Usually   5. Always

4. Which number best describes your average pain or discomfort on the days that you had it over the last week?
    1   2   3   4   5   6   7   8   9   10
    No pain   Extremely severe pain

Urination

5. How often have you had a sensation of not emptying your bladder completely after you finished urinating during the last week?
    a. Not at all.
    b. Less than one in five times.
    c. Less than half the time.
    d. About half the time.
    e. More than half the time.
    f. Almost always.

6. In the last week, how often have you had to urinate again fewer than two hours after you finished urinating?
   a. Not at all.
   b. Less than one in five times.
   c. Less than half the time.
   d. About half the time.
   e. More than half the time.
   f. Almost always.

Impact of symptoms

7. In the last week, have your symptoms kept you from your usual activities?
   a. None.
   b. Only a little.
   c. Some.
   d. A lot.

8. How much did you think about your symptoms during the last week?
   a. None.
   b. Only a little.
   c. Some.
   d. A lot.

Quality of life

9. If you were to spend the rest of your life with your symptoms just the way they have been during the last week, how would you feel about that?
   a. Delighted.
   b. Pleased.
   c. Mostly satisfied.
   d. Mixed (about equally satisfied and dissatisfied).
   e. Mostly dissatisfied.
   f. Unhappy.
   g. Terrible.

Based on Litwin MS, et al. The National Institutes of Health chronic prostatitis symptom index: development and validation of a new outcome measure. *The Journal of Urology*, 1999;162:369.

Exercise

Stretching and relaxing the lower pelvic muscles may help relieve your symptoms. Sometimes, the addition of heat with a low electric current (diathermy) may make the muscles more limber. A physical therapist can show you which exercises will benefit you the most and how to perform them. Then you can perform them regularly at home.

Biofeedback

This therapy teaches you how to control your body's responses to certain stimuli. A trained therapist will use sensors to help you get started, but over time you'll learn how to produce these positive changes yourself, such as slowing your heart rate or relaxing your muscles.

Sitz bath

From the German word *sitzen*, meaning "to sit," this type of bath involves simply sitting and soaking the lower half of your body in warm water. Many men find this therapy relieves pain and relaxes the lower abdominal muscles. Few treatments are as easy or as relaxing to do.

When prostatitis is first diagnosed, a doctor may recommend taking sitz baths two or three times a day for 30 minutes each time. For acute bacterial prostatitis, keep the water temperature below 99 F. For chronic pelvic pain, temperatures up to 115 F are fine.

Acupuncture

Acupuncture involves the insertion of very thin needles through the skin to various depths at certain points on the body. Growing evidence suggests acupuncture may help with prostatitis symptoms.

Surgery

Surgical removal of the infected portion of the prostate may be an option in severe cases of the disease when other treatments haven't worked. The most common type of surgery is transurethral resection of the prostate (TURP). A doctor may recommend the procedure when imaging tests find a visible infection (abscess) in the prostate gland.

If no abscess is found, the chance of having a positive outcome from major surgery for any type of prostatitis is quite low. For this reason, most doctors are hesitant to perform surgery for prostatitis, and generally discourage the procedure, even as a last resort.

Psychotherapy

Prostatitis is sometimes associated with reduced quality of life and depression. For these reasons, counseling may be beneficial. Cognitive behavioral therapy, in particular, which focuses on negative thought patterns, has been shown effective at addressing struggles with pain, urinary issues and sexual issues that may result from the condition.

Herbal therapies

Claims that certain natural remedies are helpful for prostatitis are unsubstantiated and await rigorous scientific study. Nevertheless, some men report that products such as saw palmetto, bee pollen extract, zinc supplements and quercetin have helped them manage their symptoms.

Keep in mind that a product's claim that it's "natural" doesn't always translate into being safe. The supplement industry is unregulated, and few well-controlled studies have been undertaken to determine efficacy or possible interactions. Always consult your doctor before using any supplement.

ANSWERS TO YOUR QUESTIONS

Does prostatitis increase my risk of cancer?

There's no evidence that acute or chronic prostatitis puts you at greater risk of prostate cancer. Prostatitis may, however, increase the level of prostate-specific antigen (PSA) in your blood. If your PSA level is elevated and you have prostatitis, it's advisable to redo the test after you've been treated with antibiotics. If you have chronic prostatitis, your doctor may test your free-PSA level (see page 30).

Can I pass a prostate infection to my partner during intercourse?

Prostatitis can result from a sexually transmitted infection, but prostatitis itself isn't contagious. Prostatitis can't be passed on through sexual intercourse, so your partner doesn't have to worry about catching an infection.

Can prostatitis make me infertile?

It may. The disease can interfere with the development of semen, making it difficult for the fluid to ejaculate properly. Because semen carries sperm, this may lower your fertility rate. A few studies indicate poor sperm quality in some men with prostatitis.

Is surgery ever used to treat the disease?

Generally, surgery isn't recommended. But if the disease has drastically affected your fertility, antibiotics aren't able to improve your symptoms or you're unable to urinate, your doctor might recommend surgery. A surgeon may try to open blocked ducts in the gland to relieve congestion and help semen flow more freely. Surgery isn't recommended for chronic nonbacterial disease.

What about saw palmetto? Can it relieve my symptoms?

Currently, there's no evidence that this popular herb relieves infection or inflammation associated with prostatitis. Furthermore, there's no evidence to show that saw palmetto is an effective treatment for noncancerous enlargement of the prostate gland (BPH). Saw palmetto is discussed in Chapter 12.

Benign prostatic hyperplasia

At birth, the prostate gland is about the size of a pea. It grows slightly during childhood, and then at puberty — generally the early teen years — it typically undergoes rapid growth. At age 20, the prostate is considered fully developed.

Most men, however, experience a second period of prostate growth a few decades later. Among men in their mid-40s, cells near the center of the prostate gland — in the transitional zone that surrounds the urethra — begin to grow.

As tissue in this zone enlarges, it often presses on the urethra and obstructs urine flow. Benign prostatic hyperplasia is the medical term for this condition. It's more commonly referred to as BPH or prostate enlargement.

BPH is common. In fact, almost all men will eventually develop the condition if they live long enough.

BPH, or prostate enlargement, isn't prostate cancer, and having BPH doesn't put you at higher risk of developing prostate cancer. Abnormal tissue growth is associated with both conditions, but the types of growth are different.

Prostate cancer develops in the outer sections of the gland, often spreading into surrounding tissue. BPH develops in the gland's interior and grows inward, constricting the urethra. Although some symptoms of BPH mimic those of cancer, BPH is a noncancerous (benign) condition. That's not to say, though, that BPH can't affect your quality of life.

Healthy prostate

Prostate enlarged by BPH

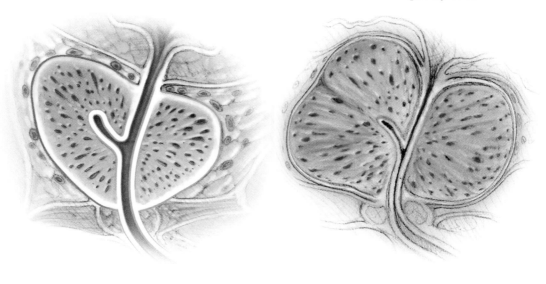

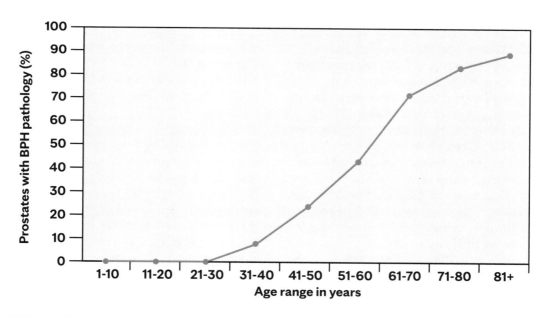

BPH prevalence BPH increases in prevalence with age but not all individuals experience signs and symptoms. Data on disease prevalence is collected at autopsy from microscopic examinations of the prostate gland.

A FACT OF LIFE

The chance that you'll develop BPH increases with age, particularly after age 40. That's when the prostate gland — primarily the gland's transitional zone — begins its second growth spurt. It's estimated that nearly 70% of men ages 60 to 70 and close to 90% of men older than age 80 have some degree of BPH.

As the prostate gland enlarges, tissue within the gland often becomes lumpy, forming characteristically uneven cell mass clusters. Smooth muscle in the prostate reacts to this buildup by constricting and tightening around the urethra, narrowing the drainage channel and obstructing urine flow from the bladder.

The exact cause of prostate enlargement is unknown, and it's likely that several factors play a role in its development. In addition to age, family history can increase your odds of developing the disease, pointing to a possible genetic link. However, genetics is thought to play a role in only a small percentage of cases. There's some evidence that obesity may increase the risk of BPH, while exercise can lower the risk. And studies show that diabetes, as well as heart disease and medications called beta blockers, might increase BPH risk.

Signs and symptoms

Signs and symptoms of BPH vary in their severity. The condition can be extremely disruptive for some men and pose few problems for others. The overall impact of BPH often is determined by the size and shape of new tissue growth, the location of the growth inside the prostate gland, and how much the bladder is affected.

A larger prostate gland doesn't always mean more severe symptoms. Symptom severity typically depends on how much the expansion of internal tissue is affecting the urethra and bladder. When symptoms are mild, many men simply live with the condition. When symptoms become annoying or more severe, men are more likely to seek medical treatment.

Common signs and symptoms of BPH include:
- A frequent or urgent need to urinate.
- Frequent urination at night (nocturia).
- Difficulty starting urination.
- A weak urine stream or a stream that stops and starts.
- Dribbling at the end of urination.
- An inability to completely empty the bladder.

At first, BPH may cause few signs and symptoms because the bladder's strong muscle can still force urine through a narrowed urethra. But the strong contractions required to empty the bladder also cause the bladder wall to thicken and become less elastic. The result is a need to urinate more often and with greater urgency.

When symptoms begin to worsen, you may start avoiding social events so that you won't face long lines at the bathroom. You may wake up tired in the morning from frequent nighttime trips to the bathroom. You may be afraid to wear light-colored pants for fear of noticeable dribbling.

Progression of the condition varies. In some cases, symptoms continue to worsen and eventually become severe. In other cases, they stay about the same or moderately worsen. In few cases, they improve over time.

For some men, the bladder may become smaller and more muscular and can no longer hold as much as it used to. This may lead to symptoms of urgency and frequency. In addition, the bladder may lose its ability to stretch, increasing pressure in the bladder and potentially causing kidney damage. For other men, the bladder stretches out, loses its muscle tone and never drains completely. A urinary catheter may be required to drain remaining urine. Urine left in the bladder can pose a serious health threat, including recurrent bladder infections and possible kidney damage.

SEEING A DOCTOR

If you're having urinary problems, discuss them with your doctor. Even if you don't find the symptoms bothersome, it's important to identify or rule out any underlying causes. A urinary problem left untreated could possibly lead to serious complications, including obstruction of the urinary tract.

At your initial visit, your doctor likely will ask about your symptoms and may conduct some basic tests to help determine if what you're experiencing is related to BPH or another condition. Instead of BPH, your symptoms could be an early warning of another condition, such as a bladder stone, bladder infection, bladder cancer, side effects of medication, heart failure, diabetes, a neurological problem, prostatitis or prostate cancer.

Expect to be asked a number of questions about your symptoms, when they developed and how often they occur. In addition, your doctor may inquire about other health problems you may have, medications you may be taking, and whether there's a history of prostate problems in your family.

In addition to information regarding your symptoms and your medical history, your checkup may include the following tests:

- A digital rectal examination to determine whether your prostate is enlarged and to help rule out prostate cancer.
- A urine test to rule out an infection or a condition that can produce similar symptoms.
- A prostate-specific antigen (PSA) blood test to help rule out cancer.

If the results of these tests suggest BPH, your doctor may request additional information and tests to help confirm the diagnosis and determine its severity.

Prostate symptom score

The American Urological Association (AUA) has developed a series of questions

PROSTATE QUESTIONNAIRE

The questions below are designed to help doctors evaluate BPH severity. It includes seven questions that are specific to your individual symptoms and a quality-of-life question that's scored separately from the seven questions. This questionnaire is known as the International Prostate Symptom Score (IPSS) or the American Urological Association symptom index.

Symptom description

Over the past month, how often have you had a sensation of not emptying your bladder completely after you finished urinating?

Over the past month, how often have you had to urinate again less than two hours after you finished urinating?

Over the past month, how often have you found you stopped and started again several times when you urinated?

Over the past month, how often have you found it difficult to postpone urination?

Over the past month, how often have you had a weak urinary stream?

Over the past month, how often have you had to push or strain to begin urination?

Over the past month, how many times did you most typically get up during the night to urinate, from the time you went to bed at night until you got up in the morning?

Scoring key
Mild symptoms: 0 to 7 total points
Moderate symptoms: 8 to 19 total points
Severe symptoms: 20 to 35 total points

Quality of life (bother score)
If you were to spend the rest of your life with these symptoms just the way they are, how would you feel about that?

Management of Benign Prostatic Hyperplasia/Lower Urinary Tract Symptoms: AUA Guideline 2021. Based on Barry MJ, et al. The American Urological Association symptom index for benign prostatic hyperplasia. American Urological Association, 1992.

	Not at all	Less than 1 time in 5	Less than half the time	About half the time	More than half the time	Almost always	Score
	0	1	2	3	4	5	_____
	0	1	2	3	4	5	_____
	0	1	2	3	4	5	_____
	0	1	2	3	4	5	
	0	1	2	3	4	5	_____
	0	1	2	3	4	5	_____
	None	**1 time**	**2 times**	**3 times**	**4 times**	**5 times**	
	0	1	2	3	4	5	_____
						Total score	
							_____
Delighted	**Pleased**	**Mostly satisfied**	**Mixed**	**Mostly dissatisfied**	**Unhappy**	**Terrible**
0	1	2	3	4	5	6

regarding specific symptoms associated with BPH, called the AUA symptom index. The International Prostate Symptom Score (IPSS) incorporates an additional question on quality of life.

For this exam, you rank how severely each symptom affects you on a scale of 1 to 5. The IPSS questionnaire includes a separate question to help gauge how much your symptoms bother you (see pages 66-67).

The separate question focuses on how you would feel about spending the rest of your life dealing with your symptoms as they are now. It's important to respond honestly. Your answer, called a "bother" score, is based on a scale from 0 to 6, with 0 being delighted and 6 being terrible. The bother score may help with deciding what, if any, treatment is appropriate.

For example, someone with moderate BPH symptoms but a low bother score may be happier with no treatment or a minimally invasive therapy rather than risking possible side effects of a more invasive procedure. On the other hand, someone with the same symptoms and a high bother score may be willing to tolerate potential side effects of a more invasive treatment to get relief.

Your responses to the symptom score will help determine your best treatment (see the diagnostic tree on page 71). If you and your doctor believe your symptoms have become too bothersome, other tests may be used to assess your condition and determine if more invasive treatment is necessary.

Voiding diary

In this diary you track the amount of fluid you drink, the number of times you urinate, and the number of times and significance of any urinary leakage over a 24- to 48-hour period.

A voiding diary is a valuable tool for assessing BPH. It may point to lifestyle changes that could improve symptoms, such as limiting how much fluid you drink, and it provides a clear record of the frequency of urination and urinary leakage.

Urodynamic studies

If there's a possibility that your symptoms are related more to the bladder than to the prostate, a series of tests may be conducted to help assess your bladder function — how much urine your bladder can hold, how much pressure builds up inside, and how full it gets when you feel the urge to urinate. Collectively, these are known as urodynamic studies.

Urinary flow test

This test measures the volume of urine expelled from the bladder per second. The results may suggest an obstruction in the urinary tract or a problem with the pelvic muscles. Keep in mind that flow rate normally decreases with age.

For the test, you urinate into a special machine in the privacy of a testing room. A flow rate of more than 15 milliliters per second (mL/s) is normal or signifies only mild disease. A rate of 10 to 15 mL/s is often associated with moderate symptoms, and less than 10 mL/s usually indicates severe BPH.

Postvoid residual test

After you finish urinating (postvoid), some urine may remain (reside) in your bladder. Retaining too much urine can cause problems. Urine backup is often a breeding ground for bacteria, leading to recurrent urinary tract infections, kidney damage and bladder stone formation.

A postvoid residual test determines how well you can empty your bladder and, if not, it measures how much urine the bladder retains. If you retain more than about ½ cup (150 to 200 milliliters), you may need further evaluation.

There are two ways to perform this test — either by inserting a flexible catheter into your bladder or by using ultrasound imaging. Ultrasound is a more common method but provides a less accurate reading.

Cystometry

For this test, a small catheter containing a pressure-measuring device called a cystometer is threaded into your bladder. Water is slowly injected into your empty bladder until you feel the need to urinate.

Also known as a pressure flow study, cystometry compares the pressure inside your bladder to the force of urine leaving your penis. It will also measure the activity of the pelvic floor muscles that keep urine from leaking.

This test helps identify obstructions that can occur from BPH or other conditions, such as bladder irritability, that can produce similar symptoms. Cystometry can also assess the function of the

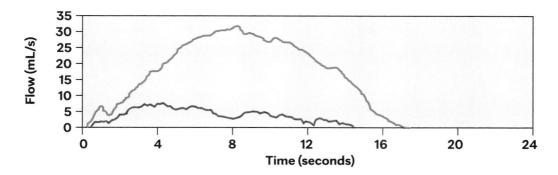

Urinary flow test The red line on this graph indicates a normal urinary flow rate, with a peak of around 30 mL/s and an average rate of approximately 20 mL/s. The blue line is a low flow rate that may indicate someone with severe BPH.

bladder muscle to determine if it has sustained significant damage due to BPH.

UroCuff test

This newer test offers a noninvasive way to measure your urine flow rate and bladder pressure. While your bladder is full, a small, inflatable cuff (similar to a blood pressure cuff) is fitted around your penis. Once the cuff is in place, you're asked to urinate into a portable commode equipped with a measuring device.

While urinating, the cuff automatically inflates until your flow of urine is interrupted and then rapidly deflates. The inflation and interruption process repeats until you're done urinating. Throughout the test, measurements are taken and recorded.

The amount of pressure applied by the cuff to stop your urine flow is equivalent to your bladder pressure. The measuring device fitted to the commode calculates the rate of urine flow. Studies indicate UroCuff test results are similar to those of conventional pressure flow studies.

Cystoscopy

A cystoscope is a flexible instrument equipped with a lens and light system that's inserted into the penis and threaded through the urethra to the bladder. It allows a doctor to see inside the urethra, including the part of the urethra surrounded by the prostate gland, and inside the bladder.

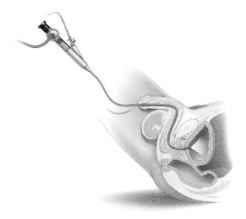

Cystoscopy A narrow, flexible tube inserted into the penis, through the urethra and to the bladder allows a doctor to examine the inside of the urethra and bladder.

The procedure can detect prostate enlargement, obstruction of the urethra or bladder neck, an anatomic abnormality, or the development of stones in your bladder. For more information on cystoscopy, see page 34.

Intravenous pyelogram or CT urography

An intravenous pyelogram is an X-ray test that helps detect urinary obstructions. For the procedure, a contrast dye that shows up on X-ray is injected into a vein and collects in the kidneys. X-ray images can reveal abnormalities in the urinary tract as the dye passes through the urinary system.

The development of newer and more detailed imaging techniques, such as computerized tomography (CT), has led to less frequent use of the intravenous

BPH DECISION TREE

Initial evaluation

- Medical history
- Prostate exam
- Symptoms score (IPSS)
- Urinalysis
- Consider urinary flow and residual testing

Complications such as urinary retention, abnormal kidney function or recurrent infections

Standard treatment
- Behavioral changes
- Medication

Alpha blocker

Lack of response or development of side effects

For average or large prostate consider adding a 5-ARI

Consider PDE-5

Lack of response or development of side effects

Discussion of surgery

Surgery

- Assess prostate size
  - Cytoscopy
  - Prostate imaging
- Consider urodynamic testing if diagnosis unclear

Large or very large prostate (> 80 cc)

- Simple prostatectomy
- Endoscopic enucleation
  - Laser; HoLEP, ThuLEP
  - Bipolar enucleation

Average prostate (30-80 cc)

- TURP
- PVP
- UroLift
- Rezum
- TUMT
- Aquablation

Small prostate (< 30 cc)

- Endoscopic enucleation
- PVP
- TUIP
- TUMT
- TURP

Concern for preservation of ejaculatory function

- UroLift (prostatic urethral lift)
- Razum (water vapor thermal therapy)

pyelogram procedure. Today, CT urography is the imaging test of choice. This technique can provide detailed cross-sectional images of the kidneys, bladder and ureters and doesn't require a contrast dye.

Prostate ultrasound

Your doctor may recommend an ultrasound exam of the prostate to adequately assess the size of your prostate gland. Size can dictate what surgical treatment would be optimal to treat your symptoms.

A prostate ultrasound is performed by placing a small probe within your rectum. Ultrasound measurements of the prostate gland are then taken to determine the size or volume of the gland. Pictures of the prostate are also taken to assess for any obvious abnormalities.

NEXT STEPS

The decision tree on page 71 is a visual guide that may help you navigate a pathway through diagnosis and possible treatment options. This guide is a general one, and your experience may differ according to your signs and symptoms, age, physical health and your doctor's recommendations.

Your decisions regarding management and treatment will be strongly influenced by how well you tolerate lower urinary tract symptoms. Each person's tolerance capacity varies. You and your doctor will want to determine your comfort range

and how you'll know that you've exceeded that range.

In the decision tree algorithm, you'll see that the IPSS questionnaire follows an initial evaluation. Mild symptoms of BPH (an IPSS score of 7 or less) may result in nothing more than careful monitoring. Moderate to severe symptoms (a score of 8 or more) usually require more tests and possible treatment.

Decades ago, the only treatment for BPH was surgery. Men generally waited until their symptoms became severe enough that surgical removal of obstructing prostate tissue became necessary. Today, other treatment options are available, including medications and less invasive therapies. They're often the first choice of treatment and can be implemented before symptoms become severe. Some men, however, may still require surgery at some point. Treatment options are discussed in detail in Chapter 5.

ANSWERS TO YOUR QUESTIONS

Are the tests to diagnose BPH painful?

Most aren't painful, but you may experience mild discomfort. Sometimes a local anesthetic is used. Advances in flexible cystoscopy have made the procedures much easier to tolerate.

Do men with larger prostates have more severe symptoms?

No. This is a common misconception. You can have a very large prostate with few or no symptoms, or a small gland with severe symptoms. That's because BPH is caused by growth in the interior of the prostate, not the outside part. Growth doesn't always affect the overall dimensions of the gland.

Does BPH increase my odds of having prostate cancer?

No evidence exists that BPH increases your risk of prostate cancer. The two conditions appear to develop independent of each other.

I've had several bladder infections in recent months. Could they be related to BPH?

There may be a relationship. BPH sometimes prevents you from completely emptying your bladder, and this can lead to infection. Talk with your doctor about testing that can determine the amount of urine left behind in your bladder after you urinate.

If I have BPH, do I have to have surgery?

If your symptoms are mild and aren't too bothersome, you and your doctor may decide to monitor your condition and see how it progresses, what's referred to as watchful waiting. If your symptoms worsen, you may opt for medication or a minimally invasive procedure to provide relief, instead of surgery. Therapies for treating BPH are discussed in the next chapter.

My father has BPH. Does that mean I'll get it, too?

Not necessarily. But because BPH does tend to run in families, your risk of developing the condition is greater than someone whose family has not experienced BPH.

Treating benign prostatic hyperplasia

Most men who seek treatment for benign prostatic hyperplasia (BPH) are bothered by persistent problems with the lower urinary tract, including frequent urination, straining to urinate and inadvertent urine leakage. Many of these problems occur because an enlarged prostate gland is blocking the urethra, causing changes in bladder function. (For more on signs and symptoms of BPH, see Chapter 4.)

Some men are willing to put up with the inconvenience of BPH rather than treat it — hoping perhaps that their symptoms will improve or not worsen. However, if your symptoms have reached a point where they're affecting your quality of life, causing anxiety and embarrassment, and preventing you from taking part in normal family life and social activities, it may be time to consult a doctor.

Another reason to not hold off treatment is that in severe cases, some men eventually lose their ability to urinate and require catheterization. Failure to treat BPH also may result in recurrent urinary tract infections, the development of bladder stones or kidney damage due to increased pressure in the bladder.

There are many treatment options for BPH. All of the treatments attempt to reduce the severity of your symptoms and restore or maintain normal functioning of your urinary tract. Each option has certain advantages and disadvantages, and each provides a different level of relief. The effectiveness of these treatments can vary and is generally dependent on factors such as your physical health, medical history and lifestyle needs.

In this chapter you'll learn about treatment options for BPH. In close partnership with your doctor, discuss the pros and cons of each therapy. Keep in mind that the severity of your symptoms and how much they bother you are key factors in determining what may be the best treatment for you. Also, depending on the size of your prostate and location of excess tissue, some options may be more appropriate than others.

It's also important that you take into account the risk of side effects and the recovery time for each treatment. Your doctor can provide you with this information and recommend the best choices.

WATCHFUL WAITING

After discussing your condition and your symptoms, you and your doctor may decide not to treat your BPH for now. Watchful waiting is generally an option for men whose symptoms are mild and not bothersome. Your doctor will still examine you regularly and monitor your condition to see if your symptoms change. Other names for this approach are observation, expectant therapy or deferred therapy.

Watchful waiting is often the preferred approach for men who don't feel their condition is interfering with daily living and who aren't bothered by getting up to urinate once or twice during the night. Watchful waiting can also be an appropriate option if your symptoms are moderate to severe, but only if you don't have complications, such as frequent bladder infections. Men who opt for watchful waiting generally aren't experiencing any complications.

The advantages of watchful waiting are that you don't have to undergo invasive treatment or deal with side effects that may evolve from treatment. Plus, watchful waiting generally doesn't cost anything more than the expense of occasional appointments with your doctor and some diagnostic tests.

The risk of this approach is that your condition could quickly and drastically worsen or that other symptoms could develop, such as acute urinary retention. These situations are uncommon, however.

Among some men who choose this approach, their symptoms stay about the same and may even improve. In most cases, symptoms tend to come and go and may gradually worsen. Some men will eventually decide to pursue more active treatment of their BPH.

While watching and waiting

A few simple lifestyle changes can often help control symptoms of BPH and prevent the condition from getting worse.
- **Empty your bladder.** Urinate all that you can when you go to the bathroom.
- **Limit beverages in the evening.** Don't drink water and other beverages for 2 to 3 hours before bedtime to help you avoid nighttime trips to the bathroom.
- **Limit caffeine and alcohol.** They can increase urine production, irritate your bladder and worsen symptoms.

- **Avoid bladder irritants.** Some men find that certain foods may worsen their symptoms. In addition to caffeine and alcohol, these include chocolate, spicy foods, acidic foods and artificial sweeteners such as aspartame.
- **Limit diuretics.** If you take diuretic medications, talk to your doctor. A lower dose, a milder form or a change in the dosage time may help. Don't stop taking your diuretics without consulting your doctor.
- **Limit decongestants and antihistamines.** These drugs tighten the sphincter muscle that controls urine flow through your urethra, making urination more difficult.
- **Schedule bathroom visits.** Try to urinate at regular times — such as every 4 to 6 hours during the day — to "retrain" the bladder. This can be especially useful if you have severe frequency and urgency.
- **Keep warm.** Colder temperatures can cause urine retention and increase the urgency to urinate.
- **Stay active.** Inactivity causes you to retain urine. Even light exercise can help relieve BPH symptoms.
- **Eat healthy.** Obesity is associated with an enlarged prostate gland.

MEDICATIONS

Taking medication to control symptoms of BPH is a common treatment approach. Medication may be prescribed to help treat moderate symptoms. It's also an option for men with mild symptoms who find their symptoms exceedingly annoying or who don't favor watchful waiting.

Three types of medications are currently used for BPH: alpha blockers, 5-alpha reductase inhibitors (5-ARIs) and phosphodiesterase-5 (PDE-5) inhibitors. Medications used to treat bladder overactivity, including anticholinergics and beta-3 adrenergic agonists, also may be used to relieve symptoms.

Medication can significantly reduce major BPH symptoms. Once you begin taking a medication that's effective, you'll need to continue taking it for life to relieve your symptoms. If you find that medications aren't helpful or they only provide modest relief, you may need to consider other approaches, including minimally invasive therapies or surgery.

Alpha blockers

This class of drugs was developed to treat high blood pressure, but these medications are also beneficial for the treatment of other conditions, including BPH. Alpha blockers relax muscles surrounding the bladder neck and muscle fibers within the prostate gland, making it easier for you to urinate.

Alpha blockers are generally the first line of drug therapy for men with BPH. They include the medications:
- Alfuzosin (Uroxatral).
- Doxazosin (Cardura).
- Silodosin (Rapaflo).
- Tamsulosin (Flomax).
- Terazosin.

Alpha blockers work quickly and effectively to relieve BPH symptoms in many men. Just a couple of weeks after taking the medication, you may already notice a much stronger urine flow and a reduced need to urinate, particularly during the night. The drugs are most effective for men with normal-size to moderately enlarged prostate glands. They may not be appropriate if you're already experiencing serious BPH complications, such as significant urine retention and frequent urinary tract infections.

Side effects are generally mild and controllable. They include headache, dizziness, stomach or intestinal irritation, and a stuffy nose. To reduce the risk of side effects, your doctor may start you out on a low dose of medication and gradually increase the dosage. If the medication causes you to feel dizzy, the best approach may be to take it before bedtime. To reduce stomach or intestinal irritation, talk to your doctor about when to take the medication, such as on a full stomach.

Some men taking alpha blockers report feeling faint when standing too quickly, what's known as orthostatic hypotension. This side effect generally improves over time. Some newer, more selective alpha blockers may cause less dizziness than older forms of the drug.

An occasionally bothersome side effect of alpha blockers is dry climax (retrograde ejaculation). This occurs when semen flows backward into the bladder instead of forward through the urethra. Although dry climax causes no harm to the body, it can be concerning for some individuals. Taking a lower dose of an alpha blocker or taking the medication every other day instead of daily may reduce this problem. The trade-off, however, may be less effective symptom relief. Certain alpha blockers also aren't recommended if you take medication for erectile dysfunction.

If you're planning to undergo cataract surgery, your doctor may recommend that you wait to begin an alpha blocker until your surgery is complete. Studies have suggested a possible link between alpha blocker use and a condition called intraoperative floppy iris syndrome (IFIS) associated with cataract surgery. It's important to let your ophthalmologist know if you take an alpha blocker.

For some men, an alpha blocker can be an especially good choice because it controls BPH and high blood pressure at the same time. This may also save you money on prescription drugs.

5-alpha reductase inhibitors (5-ARIs)

This class of medications works differently from alpha blockers. Instead of relaxing muscles in the bladder neck and prostate, 5-ARIs shrink the prostate gland or stop it from growing further. They do so by reducing the amount of dihydrotestosterone, a male hormone required for prostate gland growth.

These medications include the drugs:
- Dutasteride (Avodart).
- Finasteride (Proscar).

The medications, which can produce significant improvements in symptoms, are most effective in men with large or moderately large prostate glands. Among men with moderate to severe symptoms, 5-ARIs may decrease the occurrence of urinary retention and the need for surgery. The drugs generally aren't effective if you have a normal-size or only slightly enlarged prostate gland.

5-ARIs decrease the volume of the prostate gland, reducing pressure on the bladder neck and urethra and improving urine flow. The medications take a longer time to work than do alpha blockers. You may notice some improvement in urinary flow after a few months, but it can take six months to a year for complete results.

In most men, 5-ARIs cause limited side effects. Some men may experience impotence, decreased libido and a reduced release of semen during ejaculation. These side effects can be permanent, but for most men, they completely resolve when the medication is discontinued, or shortly thereafter.

A couple of studies raised concerns that taking a 5-ARI may increase your risk of high-grade prostate cancer. This has since been disproven, and the link was likely due to increased sensitivity of PSA testing in men on these medications, leading to better detection of cancer that was already present.

Phosphodiesterase-5 (PDE-5) inhibitors

This class of medications has been shown to regulate smooth muscle tone in the prostate gland. In particular, the Food and Drug Administration has approved a low dose of the drug tadalafil (Adcirca, Alyq, Cialis) to treat prostate enlargement. Tadalafil also is used to treat erectile dysfunction.

Tadalafil may be recommended for men with mild to moderate symptoms of BPH who also experience erectile dysfunction. Side effects are relatively rare and may include headache, flushing, stomach discomfort, nasal congestion and muscle pain. This medication isn't recommended if you have significantly decreased kidney function. Use of tadalafil in the treatment of BPH may not be covered by insurance.

Combination drug therapy

Sometimes, two medications may work better than one. Taking an alpha blocker with a 5-alpha reductase inhibitor (5-ARI) can sometimes be more effective than taking either of the drugs alone. Not only can combination therapy effectively relieve symptoms and prevent them from getting worse, but it can also lower your long-term risk of acute urinary retention or the need for surgery.

The most tested drug combination involves the medications doxazosin (Cardura) and finasteride (Proscar), but it's believed that any combination of an alpha blocker and enzyme inhibitor is effective. The side effects of combination therapy are assumed to be similar to that of each drug alone.

Men who take an alpha blocker and a 5-ARI generally get quick relief from the alpha blocker while they wait for the enzyme inhibitor to take effect — often after several months. At that time, some men may be able to discontinue use of the alpha blocker.

Alpha blockers shouldn't be taken with PDE-5 inhibitors. Studies have found that taking the two together offers no advantage. Combining an alpha blocker and a PDE-5 inhibitor also may lower blood pressure to unhealthy levels. So, don't take both medications without checking first with your doctor.

Anticholinergics

Anticholinergics relax the bladder's smooth muscle, increasing the amount of urine that your bladder can hold. The medications also reduce the pressure inside the bladder that creates urgency.

Doctors were once reluctant to prescribe anticholinergics for men with BPH out of concern that the drugs may increase the risk of acute urinary retention. However, studies suggest that using anticholinergics in combination with other BPH medications can provide symptom relief in many men without these concerns.

Anticholinergics commonly used with other BPH medications include:
• Darifenacin (Enablex).
• Fesoterodine (Toviaz).
• Oxybutynin (Ditropan).
• Solifenacin (Vesicare).
• Tolterodine (Detrol).
• Trospium (Sanctura).

Anticholinergics are available as tablets or capsules, and oxybutynin also comes as a topical patch (Oxytrol). Side effects may include dry mouth, dry eyes, constipation and drowsiness.

Beta-3 adrenergic agonist

The medication mirabegron (Myrbetriq) was developed to treat symptoms of an overactive bladder. Mirabegron also may be used in the treatment of BPH alongside other medications. When BPH is accompanied by an overactive bladder, a doctor may prescribe mirabegron to help reduce episodes of urinary frequency and urinary urgency. A side effect of mirabegron is an increase in blood pressure.

SURGERY

Not all people respond to medication. A surgical procedure is generally recommended when other treatments fail or if you have frequent urinary tract infections, bladder stones, recurrent blood in your urine or kidney damage caused by the retention of urine.

MINIMALLY INVASIVE SURGICAL THERAPIES

When medications are ineffective, minimally invasive procedures may be used to improve BPH symptoms. Many of these procedures can be performed in an office setting without the need for sedation or anesthesia. If sedation is used, it's generally a light sedation.

HERBAL THERAPIES

The Food and Drug Administration hasn't approved any herbal medications for treatment of an enlarged prostate gland.

Studies on herbal therapies as a treatment for an enlarged prostate have had mixed results. One study found that saw palmetto extract was as effective as finasteride in relieving symptoms of BPH, although prostate volumes weren't reduced. But a subsequent placebo-controlled trial found no evidence that saw palmetto is better than a placebo, an inactive substance.

Other herbal treatments — including beta-sitosterol extracts, pygeum and rye grass — have been suggested as helpful for reducing enlarged prostate symptoms. But the safety and long-term efficacy of these treatments hasn't been proved.

Make sure you learn as much as you can about the products and the benefits they claim to provide. Evaluate the benefits and risks or possible side effects. If you decide to use an herbal therapy, tell your doctor. Some herbal supplements may alter the effect of other therapies and medications. Others may create dangerous drug interactions.

For more information on herbal supplements and other alternative and complementary therapies, see Chapter 12.

Several minimally invasive therapies use a form of energy to ablate excess prostate tissue that's blocking urine flow, or they involve implantation of devices that help improve urine flow.

To determine which of the procedures may be best for you, your doctor will take into consideration several factors, including the size of your prostate, your specific symptoms and their severity, side effects of the procedures, and your personal preferences. It's important that you and your doctor discuss the pros and cons of each therapy, including the likelihood that the treatment can produce long-term relief.

Minimally invasive therapies often are more effective than medications for moderate to severe symptoms. However, just like medications, they can produce side effects, which vary with the type of treatment.

TUMT

Transurethral microwave thermotherapy (TUMT) is a computer-controlled application of microwave heat to destroy excess tissue in an enlarged prostate gland.

For the procedure, a flexible tube (catheter) is inserted through the penis and into the urethra. The catheter is equipped with a small microwave antenna that heats and destroys overgrown cells without damaging adjacent tissue. With some devices, water circulates around the antenna to protect the urethra from heat. A balloon at one end is equipped with a heat sensor to monitor the temperature.

The TUMT procedure usually takes less than an hour. Local anesthesia helps control pain, although you may feel some heat in the treatment area. You may also have a strong desire to urinate and experience bladder spasms. These responses are usually well tolerated and disappear as soon as the treatment is finished.

You generally can go home once you're able to urinate satisfactorily. However, several weeks may pass before you see a noticeable improvement in your symptoms. That's because your body needs time to break down and absorb the destroyed prostate tissue. Painful

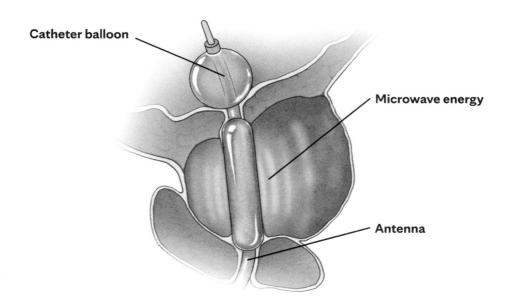

Catheter balloon

Microwave energy

Antenna

Transurethral microwave thermotherapy (TUMT) A catheter supplies computer-controlled heat to safely destroy enlarged prostate tissue. The catheter balloon at one end is equipped with a heat sensor to help control temperature.

urination may persist until the tissue is completely absorbed.

Many men require use of a urinary catheter for several days after the procedure. It's normal to experience urgency, frequent urination and small amounts of blood in your urine during the recovery period. TUMT generally doesn't produce erectile dysfunction or incontinence.

TUMT works best for men with moderately enlarged prostate glands and moderate symptoms. It doesn't work as well if the enlargement is primarily in what's called the median lobe, a posterior part of the prostate that can push against the wall of the bladder.

Because much of the prostate tissue remains after the procedure, there's a possibility you may need additional treatment in the future — either because your symptoms have returned or because they never adequately improved.

TUMT isn't recommended if you have a penile prosthesis or if you've had pelvic surgery or radiation treatments in the pelvic area. If you have a pacemaker or implanted defibrillator, consult with your cardiologist to see if the device can be deactivated before the procedure.

TUNA

This treatment, called transurethral needle ablation (TUNA), is similar to TUMT but uses high-frequency radio waves to destroy excess tissue. Use of this procedure has gradually been replaced by other treatments with better trials supporting their use and effectiveness. Evidence regarding the effectiveness of TUNA has been inconsistent. American Urological Association guidelines no longer recommend its use.

Water vapor thermal therapy

With this treatment, a special device is inserted through the penis into the urethra. It injects water vapor energy into obstructed prostate tissue to destroy (ablate) the tissue. The system that performs this procedure is known as Rezum. An advantage of the treatment is that the thermal effects of the procedure are confined to the targeted area, reducing potential damage to adjacent tissues. In addition, early studies indicate the procedure is effective and the need for repeat treatment is low.

Following treatment, you'll need to wear a urinary catheter for several days. It's normal to experience urgency, frequent urination and small amounts of blood in your urine during the recovery. Because your body needs time to break down and absorb the destroyed prostate tissue, several weeks may pass before you see a noticeable improvement in your symptoms. Urgency, frequency and painful urination may persist until the tissue is completely absorbed.

Water vapor thermal therapy can be performed in an office setting with minimal use of anesthetic or pain medications. Typically, the treatment produces few side effects, and men who have the procedure often retain erectile and ejaculatory functions.

Urethral lift

This minimally invasive therapy is marketed as the UroLift System. Under local anesthesia, a cystoscope containing a small implant device is inserted into the urethra and advanced to the area of tissue overgrowth. There, the device places an implant that lifts and holds enlarged prostate tissue that's pressing on the urethra, thereby increasing the opening of the urinary channel. The implant stays in place following the procedure, helping keep the urethra open.

With this form of treatment, there's no heating, cutting or removal of prostate tissue. Studies indicate that UroLift can significantly improve urinary symptoms and urinary flow while also preserving sexual function. However, over time, benefits of the procedure may deteriorate, and some men need additional interventions. The treatment also may not be a good option if tissue enlargement is confined to certain areas of the prostate gland where the device is less likely to be effective.

Temporary implants

Temporary implants differ from a urethral lift in that they don't remain in the urethra permanently. They're removed after a short period of time, often 5 to 7 days. The devices also work differently from a lift. One temporary implant that's been studied for BPH, called iTind, improves symptoms by creating small channels within prostate tissue through which urine can flow.

A multicenter, randomized controlled trial of iTind found the procedure to be effective and to provide rapid relief of BPH symptoms. Side effects were mild, and the procedure didn't affect sexual function.

TRANSURETHRAL SURGERY

The procedures that fit into this category usually require general anesthesia or possibly spinal anesthesia. They may be performed as an outpatient procedure in a surgery center. Sometimes an individual may need to spend one or more nights in the hospital. Transurethral procedures to treat BPH are performed with a rigid tube equipped with a lens and camera (cystoscope) that's inserted through the penis into the urethra.

TURP

Transurethral resection of the prostate (TURP) is frequently used to treat moderate to severe BPH. In fact, it's one of the more common surgeries performed on men ages 65 and older. And it's particularly effective for moderate- to large-size prostate glands for which treatment with other therapies may not be an option. There are variations of the TURP procedure, especially in relation to the type of energy source used to remove excess tissue, such as monopolar versus bipolar, but the process is similar.

With TURP, you may be placed under general anesthesia or given a spinal block. A surgeon then threads a type of cystoscope known as a resectoscope into your urethra. The resectoscope contains a light, valves for controlling irrigating fluid, and an electrical loop. The wire loop, which is heated with an electrical current, cuts away the section of the prostate gland causing symptoms and reseals opened blood vessels.

During the 60- to 90-minute operation, a surgeon removes obstructing tissue one piece at a time from inside the prostate,

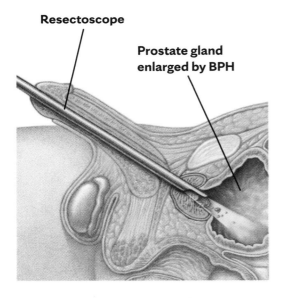

Resectoscope

Prostate gland enlarged by BPH

Transurethral resection of the prostate (TURP) With this common surgical procedure, tiny cutting tools on the resectoscope scrape away excess prostate tissue and deposit the scrapings into the bladder.

creating an interior cavity. Displaced prostate tissue is carried by the irrigating fluid into the bladder, and then is removed at the end of the procedure. A variation of this procedure is called transurethral vaporization of the prostate (TUVP). In TUVP, a button-shaped electrode is used to vaporize prostate tissue rather than cut and remove it.

TURP may require a short hospital stay after surgery. You can also expect some blood or small blood clots in your urine. You may need to wear a catheter for several days if a lot of cutting was involved, but often the catheter can be removed after a day. Many men are able to urinate on their own before leaving the hospital.

Symptom improvement should occur quickly. Most men experience stronger urine flow within a few days, and discomfort should gradually improve over 1 to 4 weeks. You can do office work in about 2 weeks and perform manual labor and resume sexual activity within 4 weeks.

TURP relieves BPH symptoms in nearly all men who undergo the procedure. It produces the greatest relief in men with larger prostate glands and more bothersome symptoms. Even men with severe bladder damage often improve after TURP.

Occasionally, TURP can cause erectile dysfunction and loss of bladder control. These complications are generally temporary. Kegel exercises (see page 168) often help restore bladder control. Other side effects of TURP are retrograde ejaculation and bladder neck contracture. The need for additional treatment is uncommon, but some men do require a second surgery, either because prostate tissue has grown back or not enough tissue was removed.

TUIP

Transurethral incision of the prostate (TUIP) involves cutting (incising) the prostate with a special instrument that's inserted through a cystoscope. Unlike TURP, no prostate tissue is removed. Instead, a surgeon cuts small grooves in the location where the urethra meets the bladder (bladder neck) as well as in the prostate gland itself. These cuts help relax the bladder neck and allow the urethra to expand slightly, reducing resistance to urine flow and making it easier for you to urinate.

The procedure typically takes 20 to 30 minutes. You may be able to return home the same day, or you may stay in the hospital overnight. Use of a catheter may be necessary for 1 to 2 days after surgery. It may take 3 to 4 weeks for symptoms to improve. Generally, you can return to work in about 2 weeks and resume sexual activity after several weeks. TUIP may be an option if you have a normal-size or minimally enlarged prostate gland.

TUIP outcomes in men who are properly selected for the procedure are, in general, similar to the outcomes for TURP. There's also less risk of complications from TUIP than from TURP, and men undergoing TUIP may be more likely to maintain ejaculation. Most men express satisfaction with TUIP, although some may experience only a small improvement in urinary flow. Additional treatment is more likely with TUIP than with TURP.

Photoselective vaporization of the prostate (PVP)

With this procedure, instead of a cutting wire, a laser is used to vaporize enlarged tissue. The PVP procedure uses energy from a potassium titanyl phosphate laser to destroy obstructing tissue. The laser creates an interior channel within the prostate that improves urine flow.

PVP takes approximately 60 to 90 minutes to perform and is generally done as an outpatient procedure. PVP has fewer side effects and a shorter recovery time than does TURP. There's usually very little bleeding, but delayed bleeding has been reported on occasion. You may experience irritation when you urinate for several weeks afterward.

PVP may be best suited for small- to medium-size prostate glands and older men with more complex medical issues. Sometimes a surgeon may combine PVP with a limited TURP procedure. For men with very large prostate glands, PVP may be done in two separate operations. A Mayo Clinic study of PVP found that most men were able to maintain symptom improvements over about a 10-year period.

A distinct advantage of PVP over other surgical procedures is that men who take

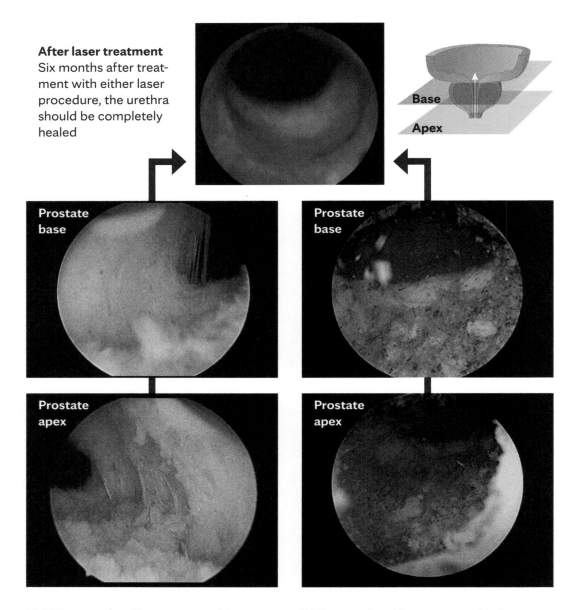

After laser treatment Six months after treatment with either laser procedure, the urethra should be completely healed

Base

Apex

Prostate base

Prostate base

Prostate apex

Prostate apex

HoLEP procedure Two cystographic images show the HoLEP enlarging a narrowed urethra (the tip of the laser is the green semicircle). Loose pieces of tissue cut from the urethra are pushed into the bladder.

PVP procedure Two cystographic images show the cavity created in the urethra by the PVP laser vaporizing excess tissue that blocks the channel. Loose, tiny fragments of tissue are visible in the images.

oral anticoagulants or antiplatelet medications can continue using them without increased risk of bleeding from the procedure.

Robotic waterjet treatment

Aquablation is the trade name for this newer procedure. It uses a heat-free waterjet controlled by robotic technology to destroy prostate tissue. Prior to activating the waterjet, a surgeon precisely maps out the area of tissue to be removed using ultrasound to image the prostate. The robot then follows the map when ablating tissue.

The procedure requires use of general anesthesia and often requires an overnight hospital stay. Robotic waterjet treatment is still fairly new, and studies haven't proved it offers advantages over other endoscopic surgical treatments. In one study, however, robotic waterjet treatment was found comparable to TURP after a period of 12 months. Side effects also were similar to those of TURP.

Transurethral enucleation

This treatment is different from other types of endoscopic surgery for BPH in that the procedures that fall into this category cleanly peel away the entire portion of the prostate gland blocking urine flow, instead of creating channels or cavities within it. It's similar to peeling an orange from the inside so that only the skin remains. The peeled prostate tissue is pushed into the bladder, where it's retrieved using a specialized instrument.

There are three treatments currently in use that fall into this category.

HoLEP

Holmium laser enucleation of the prostate (HoLEP) employs a holmium:YAG laser, which is well suited for cutting soft tissue and sealing blood vessels to reduce bleeding. HoLEP can be used on prostate glands of any size. Even extremely large glands that might otherwise require open surgery can be treated with HoLEP.

With this procedure, abnormal tissue is precisely separated from the prostate using a cutting laser. The tissue is then deposited in the bladder, leaving only a small rim of prostate tissue. Bleeding is controlled with the laser. The cut pieces are removed from the bladder with a special device called a morcellator, which grinds the tissue into smaller pieces that can be suctioned out through a cystoscope.

HoLEP is often performed as an outpatient procedure, but it may require an overnight hospital stay in some situations. A catheter typically is left in overnight and removed the next day, at which time you're asked to urinate on your own. Most men can return to their normal activities after 1 week.

Very rarely, the procedure needs to be repeated. Temporary urinary leakage after HoLEP is common, but long-term risk of urinary leakage is minimal. While HoLEP hasn't been shown to cause erectile dysfunction, retrograde ejaculation (semen entering the bladder instead of exiting the penis) may occur.

ThuLEP

Thulium laser enucleation of the prostate (ThuLEP) is similar to HoLEP but uses a thulium instead of a holmium laser. A few studies comparing the two have found the results and safety of the procedures to be similar.

Bipolar enucleation

Similar to HoLEP and ThuLEP, bipolar enucleation of the prostate removes the entire portion of the prostate gland causing the obstruction. The difference with this therapy is that it doesn't involve a laser. Instead, surgeons use a different technology — bipolar energy — to remove prostate tissue.

Studies comparing bipolar enucleation to traditional open surgery indicate comparable results and fewer complications with the enucleation procedure.

SIMPLE PROSTATECTOMY

Simple prostatectomy was once the most common treatment for an enlarged prostate gland. But with the development of newer therapies, use of more invasive surgery to treat BPH is on the decline. Today, simple prostatectomy is generally recommended when other treatments fail or in circumstances when there are complicating factors.

Simple prostatectomy is still one of the most effective and lasting ways to relieve lower urinary tract symptoms caused by BPH. However, invasive surgery is more likely to cause complications and side effects, such as infection and bleeding, than are other treatments. Invasive surgery also requires a longer recovery period, and it's not the best choice if you have a condition that would make undergoing anesthesia risky.

Simple prostatectomy is different from radical prostatectomy, which is the surgical removal of the entire prostate gland due to cancer (see page 121). Simple prostatectomy involves surgical removal of only the obstructing tissue. The procedure is usually performed in men who have greatly enlarged glands, bladder damage or other complicating factors, such as bladder stones or urethral narrowing (strictures).

With traditional open surgery, a surgeon makes an incision in your lower abdomen to reach the prostate gland rather than going up through the urethra. Only the interior portion of the gland is removed. The outer portion is left intact, much as with TURP.

The surgery is performed under general anesthesia or a spinal block and it generally requires a short stay in the hospital. You'll need to wear a catheter for approximately a week afterward. Most men can return to sedentary work in about 2 to 3 weeks, and engage in vigorous labor and sexual activity in about 6 weeks.

Nearly all men who have a simple prostatectomy experience significant symptom relief. Side effects are generally similar to those of TURP, but they may be more pronounced. There's a risk of retrograde ejaculation. However, you may be less likely to experience erectile dysfunction and incontinence than with some less invasive procedures.

Today, many medical centers now use robotics for this type of surgery. The advantage of robotic surgery is that it utilizes a couple of small incisions in the abdomen instead of a single large incision, reducing pain and shortening recovery time.

Similar to open surgery, you're under general anesthesia during the procedure. Special instruments are inserted into the small incisions. The instruments are attached to a mechanical device controlled by a surgeon who guides the instruments as they remove prostate tissue.

Some advantages of robotic surgery are reduced blood loss and more precise tissue removal to preserve urinary control. The empty cavity within the prostate gland can be reconstructed to reduce the possibility of tissue regrowth and the need for future surgeries.

Depending on which type of surgery you have — open or robotic — it may take a few weeks to several months for a full recovery. During this time, you want to avoid activities that involve lifting and those that are jarring to your pelvic area, such as operating heavy equipment or riding a bicycle.

Some degree of temporary urine leakage can be expected after surgery. To reduce leakage, you may be encouraged to do Kegel exercises (see page 168). A burning sensation at the tip of the penis also may occur, depending on the procedure performed. This also is a normal part of the healing process and improves with time. Some men experience episodes of urinary frequency and urgency because the urinary channel has been opened, and contraction of the bladder is uninhibited. This can take weeks to subside.

Constipation is sometimes a concern during recovery because you shouldn't strain your lower abdominal muscles. To prevent constipation, eat plenty of high-fiber foods, such as fruits, vegetables and grains. Fiber softens your stool and makes it easier to pass.

EMERGING TREATMENTS

No BPH treatment is perfect. They all carry some risk of side effects. For this reason, researchers continue to seek out and develop new medications and new methods for treating the symptoms of an enlarged prostate.

Medications

Experts are studying methods for improving the effectiveness and reducing the side effects of medications currently used to treat BPH. In addition, new classes of drugs are being developed that may be able to relieve lower urinary tract symptoms, either on their own or in combination with existing drugs.

Prostatic artery embolization

Prostatic artery embolization (PAE) is an outpatient procedure performed by an interventional radiologist. During the procedure, microscopic plastic beads are released into the arteries that feed the prostate gland. The beads travel through the prostatic arteries to a location in which they become lodged, obstructing the flow of blood that's causing swelling in the prostate.

A potential advantage of prostatic artery embolization is that it may cause lower rates of retrograde ejaculation or sexual dysfunction. This procedure currently isn't recommended by the American Urologic Association and is generally reserved for men who aren't candidates for surgery due to existing health conditions.

Interstitial laser therapy

Interstitial laser therapy (ILT) destroys excess prostate tissue with laser energy. A specially designed fiber-optic device is inserted through a cystoscope and into the urethra. The device punctures through the wall of the urethra into areas of the prostate containing overgrown tissue. Once inside the prostate, the laser is activated to heat and destroy the tissue.

Several punctures are usually needed to treat the entire area that's affected.

Interstitial laser therapy is thought to be most effective for men with normal-size or moderately enlarged prostates with mild to medium changes in bladder function.

FACTORS TO CONSIDER

BPH can be treated in many ways, and each option has its distinct advantages and disadvantages. No one can predict which treatment will work best for you. The course of treatment you decide on is the one that you and your doctor feel is right after careful consideration.

Keep in mind, the studies comparing the pros and cons of different treatments look at large populations of men. But you are one man — with your own concerns, health history, and levels of tolerance and discomfort. You must balance what you read with how you feel.

As you mull over the treatment options, it may help you to consider these key decision points and discuss them with your doctor.

How severe are your symptoms?

If the symptoms don't bother you and your condition isn't causing complications, you can probably wait to see if the symptoms improve or worsen. On the other hand, if you have severe symptoms, organ damage or complicating factors, such as frequent urinary infections, bleeding or bladder stones, you may need surgery.

Treating anything in between depends on personal preference. Will you settle for small improvements, or are you hoping for more noticeable changes in your symptoms? Do you want immediate relief, or can you wait? Are you willing to take medication daily? Will you tolerate some side effects?

How bothered are you by your symptoms?

This is a key question in the decision process that only you can respond to. You may have strong urinary tract symptoms caused by an enlarged prostate, but you may not be as bothered by them as another man with only moderate symptoms. If you're not bothered by your symptoms, there may be little or no benefit in treating them.

As a rule of thumb, for men with mild symptoms, active surveillance is often the best approach. Men with moderate symptoms are often candidates for medication. Men with severe symptoms are typically candidates for minimally invasive treatments or surgery.

Are your symptoms getting worse?

Symptoms often come and go in men with mild to moderate BPH. But over the long term, they will tend to worsen. If you notice your symptoms getting worse, talk to your doctor.

One way to gauge if your symptoms are getting worse is to periodically complete the prostate symptom index (see pages 66-67) and evaluate any changes in your symptoms.

How big is your prostate gland?

Some BPH treatments are best suited for large prostates, while others are more effective for smaller or average-size prostates.

Treatments that may be better for small prostates include:
- Alpha blockers.
- Transurethral microwave thermotherapy (TUMT).
- Transurethral incision of the prostate (TUIP).
- Transurethral resection of the prostate (TURP).
- Photoselective vaporization of the prostate (PVP).
- Holmium laser enucleation of the prostate (HoLEP).
- Thulium laser enucleation of the prostate (ThuLEP).

For average-size prostates, treatment options generally include:
- Alpha blockers.
- 5-alpha reductase inhibitors (5-ARIs).
- Prostatic urethral lift.
- Transurethral microwave thermotherapy (TUMT).
- Water vapor thermal therapy.
- Transurethral resection of the prostate (TURP).
- Photoselective vaporization of the prostate (PVP).

- Robotic waterjet treatment.
- Holmium laser enucleation of the prostate (HoLEP).
- Thulium laser enucleation of the prostate (ThuLEP).

Therapies that are better suited for large or very large prostates include:
- 5-alpha reductase inhibitors (5-ARIs).
- Transurethral enucleation of the prostate (HoLEP, ThuLEP, bipolar enucleation).
- Open and robotic simple prostatectomy.

What's your age?

The best treatment for a man in his 50s may not be the best for a man in his 80s. If you're younger, you may choose one of the minimally invasive treatments that provide long-term benefits, even if they don't provide immediate relief.

If you're older, immediate symptom relief provided by alpha blockers or surgery might be more important to you than long-term benefits. On the other hand, the older you are, the less suited you are to tolerate surgery. You may also recover from it more slowly.

How healthy are you?

If you have other serious health problems, you may not be a good candidate for surgery or recover from it as quickly. Surgery generally isn't recommended if you have:

- Uncontrolled diabetes.
- Cirrhosis of the liver.
- Serious lung, kidney or heart disease.
- A major psychiatric disorder.
- A short life expectancy.

Some people aren't good candidates for medication because they don't tolerate a specific drug or class of medications.

Do you want to father more children?

If you want to father children, avoid therapies that may cause infertility. TURP, TUIP, HoLEP and simple prostatectomy are the BPH treatments that are most likely to cause retrograde ejaculation, in which semen backs up into your bladder instead of ejaculating from your penis. Less often, laser surgery and alpha blockers cause this problem. Unlike erection problems, which may be temporary, retrograde ejaculation is often permanent.

Procedures such as water vapor thermal therapy and a urethral lift may be recommended because they're unlikely to cause retrograde ejaculation or erectile dysfunction.

How sexually active are you?

Surgery may damage nerves or blood vessels located next to the prostate gland, causing permanent erection problems. Often, however, erection problems are temporary and normal sexual function, including the ability to have an erection and orgasm, returns after a few months.

Erection problems — even short-lived — are a concern for many men. Discuss this issue with your doctor before surgery.

Do the benefits outweigh the risks?

TURP — a surgical procedure — is still widely used to treat BPH despite the risk of more serious side effects because it's excellent at relieving symptoms, it relieves them quickly, and it rarely requires a second treatment.

Minimally invasive therapies are a trade-off alternative to surgery. They don't work quite as well or as fast as surgery does, and they're more likely to require retreatment after several years. On the other hand, they're less likely to cause serious side effects, and they generally cost less.

As for medication, alpha blockers and enzyme inhibitors appear to offer long-term benefits, especially when used in combination. But they can cause side effects, you have to take them indefinitely, and the costs add up.

How long will it take to recover?

Recovery time varies with the treatment. If you choose medication, you don't have to worry about being laid up or missing work.

Minimally invasive surgical therapies are often performed on an outpatient basis, and you may need to restrict activities for a limited time. Many transurethral surgical procedures also are performed on an outpatient basis, but occasionally require an overnight stay. A urinary catheter is left in place temporarily after most endoscopic procedures. You'll want to avoid strenuous activity and heavy lifting for 1 to 6 weeks, depending on the procedure. Discuss the need for any restrictions with your doctor before surgery.

More invasive procedures for BPH, such as simple prostatectomy, may require a 3- to 5-day hospital stay. You may need to take up to a month off work, and for up to 6 weeks you'll need to avoid heavy lifting, jarring your lower pelvic area or straining your lower abdominal muscles. Recovery may be a bit quicker with robotic surgery.

How experienced is your doctor?

Make sure that the treatment you and your doctor decide on is the best one for you — which is not necessarily the treatment your doctor has the most experience with. At the same time, in general, the more experience your doctor has with a particular therapy, the lower the risk of side effects and the greater your chances of a noticeable improvement.

ANSWERS TO YOUR QUESTIONS

Can treatment for BPH reduce my risk of getting cancer?

It may, depending on the treatment you receive. A major study showed that taking finasteride (Proscar) prevented or delayed the onset of prostate cancer by 25% in men ages 55 and older. However, the same study showed that finasteride may contribute to an increased risk of sexual side effects.

Other BPH treatments don't reduce the risk of prostate cancer, with the exception of complete prostate removal (radical prostatectomy). Even if you're being treated for BPH, you still need to continue regular prostate exams to screen for cancer. Some treatments for BPH, however, can identify cancer in its early stages. For example, unsuspected cancer is found during TURP in about 10% to 15% of men.

Is the medication finasteride the same drug that I see advertised for hair growth?

Yes. Finasteride is used to treat both BPH and hair loss. When prescribed to manage BPH, finesteride is sold under the brand name Proscar. When used to treat hair loss, it's sold as Propecia. The only difference is the dose. Proscar, for BPH, comes in a 5-milligram (mg) tablet. Propecia, for hair growth, comes in a 1-mg tablet.

If the first treatment option I choose doesn't work, can I try another?

Absolutely. Conservative options, such as medication, are often the first choice of many men and their doctors. If conservative options don't produce satisfactory results, then you can move on to more invasive treatments.

Should I get a second opinion before deciding on a treatment?

Not necessarily. It depends on the confidence you have in your doctor and the therapeutic option that you choose.

If you select a more conservative treatment, such as medication, or a minimally invasive therapy, a second opinion may not be necessary. It's also important that your doctor has adequate experience with the therapy being recommended that you feel comfortable with the decision. If you don't feel comfortable with your doctor's recommendation, it might be a good idea to consult another doctor.

After surgery or a minimally invasive procedure, are there steps that I can take to reduce my risk of complications?

Your care provider may recommend that you avoid heavy lifting and exercises that strain the groin or lower abdominal area for a couple of weeks to a couple of months after the procedure. How long these restrictions are in place will depend, in part, on the procedure that you have.

Other steps that you can take to promote a healthy recovery and reduce complications include staying hydrated, eating a healthy diet, avoiding stimulants such as caffeine, alcohol and nicotine, and getting regular exercise.

If you have questions about your follow-up care, don't be afraid to contact a member of your health care team.

Keep in mind that it's normal to experience urgency, frequent urination and small amounts of blood in your urine during the recovery period. Contact your doctor if the blood in your urine is thick like ketchup, the bleeding appears to be worsening or your urine flow is blocked. Blood clots can block urine flow.

PART 3

Prostate cancer

Learning you have cancer

6

Prostate cancer is the most diagnosed cancer in men in the United States, aside from certain skin cancers, which are typically less life-threatening. The American Cancer Society estimates that 268,490 new cases of prostate cancer will be diagnosed in 2022, and more than 34,000 men will die of the disease. Prostate cancer ranks as the second leading cause of cancer deaths among American men, after lung cancer.

Approximately 1 in 8 men will be diagnosed with prostate cancer in their lifetimes. As you age, your risk of prostate cancer increases. It's estimated that by age 50, about one-third of men have some cancerous cells in their prostate glands. By age 80, this increases to about three-quarters of all men. The average age of diagnosis for prostate cancer is 66.

Not all cancers act the same. Typically, prostate cancer grows slowly and remains confined to the gland, where it doesn't cause serious harm. Often, the cancer produces no signs or symptoms until it becomes more advanced. Some men may live long, healthy lives without ever knowing of a problem, many times dying of something unrelated to prostate cancer.

Other times, the cancer produces signs and symptoms. For example, there may be an increase in prostate-specific antigen (PSA) levels in your blood, or a firm nodule may be detected during a digital rectal exam (DRE). These results generally warrant further evaluation and potential treatment.

Some forms of prostate cancer can be extremely aggressive, and these cancers

WHAT IS CANCER?

Cancer is a disease caused by abnormal cells that divide and grow uncontrollably. These cells can spread to normal tissue and destroy normal cell function. If not detected early, cancer often becomes life-threatening.

Cancer begins with damage (mutation) to the DNA in certain body cells. DNA contains a set of instructions that tells your cells how to grow, divide, develop specialized functions and eventually die. Normal cells frequently develop DNA mutations but also have the ability to repair most of the damage. If the cells can't make the repairs, they typically die.

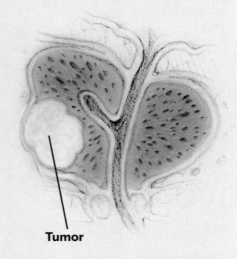

Tumor

The overall health of your body depends, in part, on this delicate balance between cell growth and development and the natural process of cell death (apoptosis). Sometimes, however, the process breaks down and certain mutations aren't repaired or eliminated. When that happens, cells can grow without restraint and become cancerous. Mutations also cause these cells to live beyond their normal life span.

In some cancers, but not all, the abnormal cells form small clusters (nodules) that develop into more densely packed, hard tumors. Cancerous cells can invade and destroy normal cells, either by growing directly into adjoining organs and tissues — referred to as local-regional spread — or by traveling to another part of your body through your bloodstream or lymphatic system, called metastatic spread.

quickly spread to other parts of the body. On average, an American male has about a 3% risk of dying of prostate cancer. This is because treatment of the disease can be very effective when steps are taken early and because other illnesses may ultimately cause death before the cancer itself.

The reasons why some prostate cells become cancerous and others don't, and why certain types of prostate cancer behave differently from others are unknown. Research suggests a combination of factors may play a role, including family history, ethnicity, hormones, diet and environment. (See "Are you at risk?" beginning on page 17.)

However, this much is clear: Most prostate cancer that's detected while the cancer is still confined to the prostate gland can be cured. It's after the cancer has spread to nearby organs that treating the disease becomes more difficult — but not impossible.

Put simply, your goal — just like your doctor's — is to catch prostate cancer early. That gives you more treatment options and a much better chance of survival and preserving your quality of life.

SIGNS AND SYMPTOMS

One thing that makes diagnosing and treating prostate cancer challenging is that typically there are no early warning signs. The condition may easily go undetected until the cancer spreads beyond the prostate gland, at which point it becomes much harder to treat.

Another challenge: When signs and symptoms of advanced prostate cancer do develop, it's very easy to attribute them to another disorder. For example, many symptoms are similar to those you would experience with benign prostatic

hyperplasia (BPH), a noncancerous condition (see Chapter 4).

Signs and symptoms of prostate cancer that can result when a tumor presses on the bladder or urethra include:
• Sudden need to urinate.
• Difficulty starting to urinate.
• Pain during urination.
• Weak urine flow and dribbling.
• Intermittent urine flow.
• Sensation that your bladder isn't empty.
• Frequent urination at night.
• Blood in your urine.

Other signs and symptoms that may signal prostate cancer include:
• Dull pain in your lower pelvic area.
• General pain in the lower back, abdomen, hips or upper thighs.
• Painful ejaculation.
• Painful bowel movements.
• Loss of appetite and weight.
• Incontinence.
• Lethargy.

Although these signs and symptoms are often an indicator of noncancerous conditions, it's important to contact your doctor for an evaluation so that, whatever the problem is, it can be treated.

SCREENING AND DIAGNOSIS

Because prostate cancer frequently doesn't cause signs and symptoms, regular screening tests are available for detecting cancer in its early stages. Men who choose to have prostate screening after discussing the benefits and risks of testing with their doctors usually begin in their 50s. But evidence suggests that establishing an earlier baseline (between ages 40 and 50) can predict later development of aggressive prostate cancer.

Routine screening tests include a digital rectal exam and the PSA test. For a description of these procedures, see pages 22-25.

By themselves, these screening tests are simple — though they're not foolproof. However, because a digital rectal exam and a PSA test detect cancer in different ways, comparing the results of the two may correct some oversight of the individual tests. That makes it more likely to catch the cancer at an early stage.

ELEVATED PSA AND USE OF MRI

MRI of the prostate has emerged as a very promising tool in evaluating men with elevated PSA levels. Previously, individuals with elevated PSA levels often proceeded directly to biopsy to determine whether the increase in PSA was related to cancer. This resulted in many men receiving biopsies who didn't have cancer and whose PSA was elevated for other reasons. The straight-to-biopsy strategy also led to the overdiagnosis of low-grade prostate cancer, defined as a Gleason score of 6. (You can read about Gleason scores beginning on page 103.) Low-grade cancers often don't require any treatment, meaning that many men underwent unnecessary testing and intervention, and they may have experienced unwarranted anxiety.

Use of MRI early in the diagnostic process has led to more selective use of biopsy procedures to identify men with higher-risk prostate cancers who may require treatment. And it has significantly reduced the rate of unnecessary biopsies in men with no prostate cancer or low-grade prostate cancer. In addition, use of MRI has increased biopsy accuracy by allowing doctors to focus on spots identified on the MRI that are more likely to be cancerous.

Like any test, however, MRI isn't 100% accurate. In approximately 10% of cases, MRI will miss a clinically significant cancer — a Gleason score of 7 or higher.

Whether you have an MRI before undergoing a prostate biopsy will ultimately depend on several factors, including your PSA value, suspicion of prostate cancer, doctor preference, as well as having insurance that covers use of MRI prior to biopsy.

More recently, use of magnetic resonance imaging (MRI) is being incorporated into the evaluation of men with elevated PSA levels prior to undergoing a prostate biopsy. An MRI can identify lesions or spots in the prostate that may be cancer and help guide the decision of whether to have a biopsy.

Biopsy

During a biopsy procedure, small tissue samples are removed from the gland and analyzed to determine if cancer cells are present. A biopsy is the only definitive way to diagnose prostate cancer.

For the procedure, a doctor inserts an ultrasound probe into your rectum. Images produced by the probe help visually guide the procedure. Once the probe is in place, thin sections of tissue are removed from the prostate gland using a spring-powered instrument called a biopsy gun, which propels a fine, hollow needle into the gland.

Most often, the biopsy needle is inserted through the rectum wall into your prostate (transrectal biopsy). Your doctor may choose to use an alternative technique called transperineal biopsy. With this method, the needle is inserted through the perineum, the area of skin between the rectum and the scrotum (see the illustration on page 102).

Transperineal biopsy is becoming more common because of a major advantage: It reduces the risk for a potentially life-threatening infection (sepsis) because it doesn't contaminate the prostate with material from the rectum. For a transperineal biopsy, an ultrasound probe still is placed in the rectum.

If an abnormal area is identified on the ultrasound image, your doctor will biopsy that area, and take approximately 12 tiny samples from various parts of the prostate gland. This is referred to as a systematic biopsy, or sextant biopsy. Most of the samples are taken from the outer portion of the gland (peripheral zone), where cancer most often develops. (See the prostate zone diagram on page 14.) Sometimes, samples are also taken from the interior of the gland (transitional zone).

MRI may also be used during a prostate biopsy, providing a more detailed picture of abnormal areas in need of additional analysis. MRI-fusion biopsy has shown considerable promise in the detection of prostate cancers that may warrant treatment, especially among men with previously negative biopsies who are experiencing an unexplained increase in PSA.

In preparation for a biopsy, you're given local anesthesia to reduce or eliminate any discomfort. Most men have only mild discomfort during the procedure and usually don't require pain medication afterward.

You may be given an enema to help empty your colon to aid in visualization and to reduce your risk of infection during the biopsy procedure. Antibiotics taken before the biopsy can further reduce the risk of infection.

Common side effects of a biopsy include a small amount of rectal bleeding with a transrectal biopsy, and blood in your urine for 1 to 2 days. Blood may appear in your semen, giving it a pink tint, for weeks to months afterward. Infection after a biopsy is also possible, although severe infection is uncommon. It's also common to experience temporary slowing of your urine stream, and there's a small chance of urinary retention requiring temporary catheter placement.

Biopsy samples are sent to a pathologist, a doctor who specializes in diagnosing tissue abnormalities. A pathologist determines whether cancer is present in the samples and if present, how aggressive the cancer is.

Samples taken during a biopsy can also identify specific cells that may be associated with later development of prostate cancer. Known as prostatic intraepithelial neoplasia (PIN), these abnormal cells

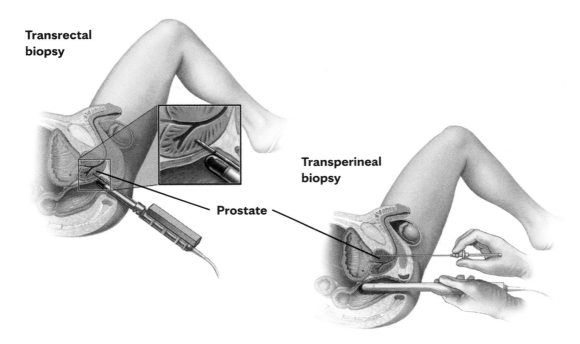

Transrectal biopsy A biopsy needle is inserted into the rectum. The needle passes through the rectal wall and into suspicious areas within the prostate gland. Small sections of tissue are removed for analysis.

Transperineal biopsy The procedure is similar, but the biopsy needle is inserted through the perineal skin, not the rectum, into the prostate gland. The perineum is the area between the anus and the genitals.

were previously thought to be early indicators of cancer — the early stages of a cell turning cancerous. Findings now suggest that the risk of prostate cancer among men with PIN is similar to that for men with noncancerous findings on a biopsy. However, men with multiple areas of high-grade PIN on a biopsy may require more careful observation.

For men whose biopsies show atypical small acinar proliferation (ASAP), there's a slightly higher probability of finding prostate cancer on a later biopsy. If you have ASAP, your doctor may closely monitor your PSA levels and may recommend a later biopsy or prostate MRI, usually within one year.

GRADING CANCER

When a biopsy confirms the presence of cancer, the next step, called grading, determines if it's a slow- or fast-growing form. A pathologist studies your tissue samples under a microscope, comparing the cancer cells with healthy prostate cells. The more the cancer cells in your sample differ from healthy cells, the more aggressive your cancer is and the more likely it is to spread quickly.

The pathologist will assign numerical grades to the cancer cells, indicating how aggressive they are. But a single grade cannot reflect the complexity of this disease. Cancer cells often vary in size and shape throughout a single sample, with some cells appearing more aggressive and other cells appearing less aggressive.

When there's variance, the pathologist will identify the two most numerous types of cancer cells in your sample, based in part on how the cells have fused or formed into scattered masses. Both types are assigned a grade, based on what's known as the Gleason grading scale. Using the sum of these two numbers, the cancer is then assigned a Gleason grade group.

For example, the most common type of cancer cell in a biopsy sample may be a grade 4 cancer, while the second most common is a grade 3. The two numbers are added together to determine a total Gleason score — in this case, 4 + 3 equals a score of 7 and a Gleason grade group of 3.

In comparison, if the most common type in the sample was a grade 3 cancer and the second most common type was a grade 4, the two numbers added together

GLEASON SCORES

Gleason score	Gleason grade group
3 + 3	1
3 + 4	2
4 + 3	3
4 + 4	4
4 + 5, 5 + 4, 5 + 5	5

THE GLEASON GRADING SCALE

The Gleason grading scale runs from 3 to 5, with 3 being the least aggressive form of cancer cell and 5 being the most aggressive form. Previous designations — Gleason grades 1 and 2 — are no longer used. These patterns of cells are thought to represent variations in typical prostate tissue.

Grade 3. Cancer cells are varied in size and shape, unevenly spaced, with some cells fused together into large, oddly shaped clumps.

Grade 4. Many cancer cells are fused into clumps that are scattered haphazardly and are invading nearby tissue.

Grade 5. Most cancer cells have gathered into large, scattered masses that have invaded nearby tissues and organs.

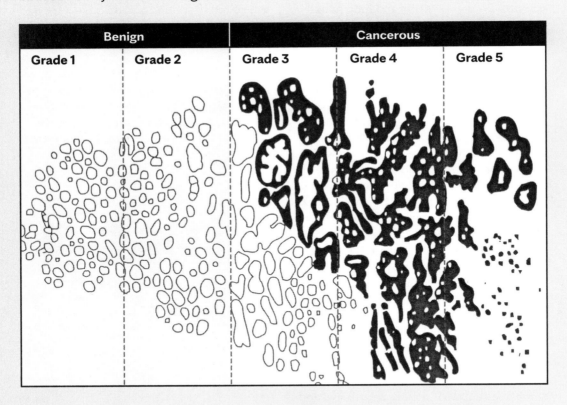

Based on Epstein JI, et al. The 2005 International Society of Urological Pathology (ISUP) Consensus Conference on Gleason Grading of Prostatic Carcinoma. The American Journal of Surgical Pathology. 2005;29:1228.

would appear as 3 + 4, which also equals 7 but which equates to a Gleason grade group of 2.

The Gleason score is a very important factor in determining how aggressive prostate cancer is — in other words, the likelihood of cancer spreading outside the prostate gland — and disease prognosis. Your Gleason score helps your doctor determine the best course of treatment for you.

Scoring can range from 6 (nonaggressive cancer) to 10 (very aggressive cancer). The lower the score, the better. A score of 6 usually indicates a low-risk cancer with a minimal chance of spreading. A score of 7 indicates a moderately aggressive cancer. Scores at the high end of the scale, from 8 to 10, mean the cancer is fast growing and has a greater chance of spreading.

Gleason grade group designations further distinguish which prostate cancers may be aggressive, with a 1 having a low risk for cancer spread and a 5 a high risk of spread.

BIOPSY TISSUE GENOMIC TESTING

A Gleason score is a useful tool for predicting the aggressiveness of your cancer. However, it doesn't always tell the whole story. This is where genomic testing may come into play.

Today, tests are available that can help your doctor decide whether your cancer is one that should be treated or if active surveillance is a viable option. Many tests are being investigated for this purpose. The following are currently approved by the FDA.

Oncotype DX

This test identifies biomarkers that predict spread (metastasis) and cancer recurrence. The absence of these markers in a biopsy specimen points to a lower-risk cancer that may only require surveillance. The results of this test are reported as a Genomic Prostate Score (GPS).

Prolaris

This test functions much like Oncotype DX, measuring how fast your tumor is growing. By analyzing certain genetic markers, your Prolaris score helps your doctor recommend the best course of treatment. The test can also be used after prostatectomy to estimate the risk of recurrence.

Decipher

This test can be used at the time of biopsy to determine whether you are a candidate for active surveillance or should undergo treatment. It's also useful for men who've undergone surgery to remove the prostate gland (radical prostatectomy). It measures certain biomarkers in the removed prostate tumor to determine the activity of genes involved in cancer progression. This helps determine the likelihood that the cancer will spread in the next 5 years.

While genomic testing may be a beneficial resource, it can be expensive, and insurance coverage varies.

ADDITIONAL TESTS

Depending on your doctor and your cancer, one or more of the following tests may be performed to help determine whether your cancer has spread. Many men don't require additional tests and can proceed with treatment based on the characteristics of their tumors and the results of their PSA tests.

Ultrasound

Ultrasound imaging may be used to determine the size and shape of your prostate. It's generally done at the time of biopsy to help guide the procedure. It's rarely performed after you've been diagnosed with prostate cancer. Typically, the test takes about 30 minutes or less. For more on ultrasound, see page 35.

Bone scan

A picture is taken of your skeleton to help determine if cancer has spread to your bones. A bone scan isn't necessary in evaluating all cases of prostate cancer, and generally isn't performed when there's little reason to suspect cancer spread.

Typically, bone scans are used in men with Gleason scores of 4 + 3 and higher, and in men who have symptoms of bone metastasis, such as bone or back pain, high blood calcium levels or other abnormal lab results. For more on this imaging procedure, see page 44.

Chest X-ray

An X-ray image can show if the cancer has spread to your lungs. Although prostate cancer usually doesn't spread this far, studies have shown that lung metastases have developed in many people with more advanced prostate cancer. For more on the X-ray procedure, see page 36.

Computerized tomography

Commonly referred to as a CT scan, this imaging procedure produces cross-sectional images of body tissue — each scan representing a thin slice of your body. A computer gathers the cross-sectional images to form a detailed 3D picture, allowing a doctor to view your prostate or other parts of your body from any angle (see page 38).

A CT scan isn't necessary in every case of prostate cancer. As with a bone scan, your doctor may decide to order a CT scan only if there's reason to suspect that the cancer has spread from the prostate to surrounding areas. It's most often used in men with a Gleason score of 4 + 4 and higher, and some cancers with a Gleason score of 4 + 3.

On a CT scan, areas of new bone growth — from cancer, fracture, arthritis or infection — appear denser than old bone. In addition, a CT scan can identify enlarged lymph nodes. When cancer begins to spread, one of the first places it goes to is your lymph nodes. In prostate cancer, this is usually the pelvic lymph nodes. The lymph nodes trap and try to destroy abnormal cells, causing the nodes to swell. Eventually, the nodes are overwhelmed by the cancer.

What a CT scan can't do is distinguish between cancer and another condition as the cause of lymph node swelling. And it can't detect microscopic levels of cancer in normal-size nodes.

Magnetic resonance imaging

Commonly referred to as MRI, it produces a detailed, 3D picture of your body. Instead of using X-rays and dyes, MRI uses magnets and radio waves to generate images (see page 40).

An MRI is commonly used to diagnose cancers that have spread outside the prostate gland, including to lymph nodes and bone. An MRI offers better detail of structures around the prostate than does a CT scan, such as whether cancer has spread beyond the prostate capsule into nearby structures like the seminal vesicles or neurovascular bundles, the bladder, or less often, the rectum.

MRI also is useful for confirming limited and nonaggressive disease in men who choose active surveillance and for identifying sites of recurrent cancer after treatment.

Lymph node biopsy

A biopsy is the best way to confirm that cancer has spread to nearby lymph nodes in the pelvic region. A biopsy is usually performed by a specially trained radiologist, in which a long needle is inserted through the skin into a lymph node. The sample is sent to a pathologist for analysis.

Lymph node biopsy is most often performed when a CT scan or MRI suggests lymph node involvement. Biopsy results can provide a clearer picture of the extent of cancer and increase certainty about treatment decisions. Not everyone needs a lymph node biopsy, particularly if your doctor strongly suspects node involvement based on PSA scores and imaging tests. With the advent of highly sensitive tests such as the PSMA PET scan, suspicious lymph nodes found on CT imaging can be further evaluated for metastasis with a PET scan rather than a biopsy.

Positron emission tomography

This form of nuclear imaging measures certain chemical processes taking place in your body. Positron emission tomography (PET) can help doctors distinguish between the normal and abnormal function of different organs and tissues.

When a PET scan is performed on the prostate gland, you'll receive an injection of a radioactive tracer combined with choline, PSMA or another substance, which is either absorbed by prostate cancer cells or sticks to the surface of the prostate cells. A PET scanner detects the emission of this radioactive energy (positrons). The number of positrons detected indicates how much of the tracer was absorbed by the cells. Cancer cells absorb more of these compounds and appear on the scan as bright, intense colors (hot spots). In this way, the scan can show where cancer cells are in your body (see pages 45-46).

A PET scan is routinely integrated with a CT scan to more precisely determine where cancer cells are located. Results of a PET scan help your doctor determine possible spread of cancer outside your prostate gland or assess how your cancer is responding to treatment. A PET scan must be interpreted carefully by doctors trained specifically in this technique.

Conventional PET scans that use radioactive sugar or glucose (FDG-PET) aren't effective for evaluating prostate cancer. Instead, radiotracers such as choline (choline C-11 PET); gallium (Ga 68 PSMA-11 PET), which targets a prostate cancer protein called prostate-specific membrane antigen, or PSMA; and fluciclovine (F 18 PET) are used.

PET scans of the prostate are used most often when it's suspected that cancer has recurred after treatment — usually when cancer blood tumor markers, such as PSA, are rising. However, PSMA PET scans are now also being used for initial staging of prostate cancer.

In the case of cancer recurrence, particularly when PSA values are low, locating the cancer can be difficult. The role of PET scans in identifying recurrent cancer is discussed further in Chapter 8.

CANCER STAGING

Grading indicates the aggressiveness of the cancer. Staging determines if or how far the cancer has spread. Your doctor assigns a stage to your cancer based on careful study of all your test results.

This step is crucial because cancer that's confined to the prostate has a very high cure rate. Once the cancer spreads beyond the prostate, the survival rate declines. The staging designation communicates to you and your health care team how advanced your cancer is.

Some men find staging information helpful for discussing treatment options with their doctors. Other men find the information overwhelming. If you have questions about your diagnosis or cancer stage, discuss them with your doctor.

TNM system

The TNM system is the most commonly used staging system for cancer in the United States. When a pathologist sends your doctor a report that stages your cancer, the report will include three capital letters — T, N and M.
- **T** stands for tumor and indicates the extent of the cancer in and adjacent to the prostate gland.
- **N** stands for nodes (lymph nodes) and indicates whether the cancer has spread to nearby lymph nodes.

- **M** stands for metastasis, the medical term for cancer that has spread to other tissues or organs, such as bone, distant lymph nodes or the lungs.

Each letter is followed by a number and perhaps another letter in small type. The numbers range from 0 to 4 and represent the extent of the tumor. The small letters used are a, b and c and indicate the location of the cancer.

Once the T, N and M results are known, the cancer is assigned one of four stages (see the illustration on pages 110-111).

Stage I

This signifies very early cancer that's confined to small particles in the prostate that can't be felt during a digital rectal exam. This stage is most commonly found as a result of an elevated PSA, but it might also be observed during a procedure for BPH.

Stage II

The cancer is large enough to be felt during a digital rectal exam screening test, but it remains confined to the prostate gland.

Stage III

The cancer has spread beyond the prostate to the tissue surrounding the prostate or the seminal vesicles, rectum, bladder or pelvic side wall.

Stage IV

This represents advanced cancer that has spread to the lymph nodes, bones, lungs or other organs.

Risk group assessment

Risk group systems are sometimes used to help determine if the cancer has spread outside the prostate gland. This system uses your PSA level, biopsy results including Gleason score and the T stage of the cancer to determine your risk. Your placement into one of these risk groups can help determine the best treatment approach for you. (See pages 103-105 for an explanation of the Gleason score.)

Low-risk group

It includes the following: PSA less than or equal to 10 and Gleason score 6 and cancer stage T1 to T2a. If you meet certain criteria, you might be considered very low risk. Criteria include PSA less than or equal to 10 and Gleason score 6 and cancer stage T1c and fewer than three biopsy cores positive, with 50% or less of each biopsy core containing cancer. PSA density (PSA divided by prostate volume) must also be less than 0.15.

Intermediate-risk group

Placement into this group involves a PSA between 10 and 20 and/or Gleason score of 7 and/or cancer stage less than T2c.

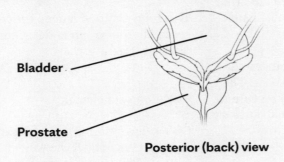

Bladder

Prostate

Posterior (back) view

Stage I

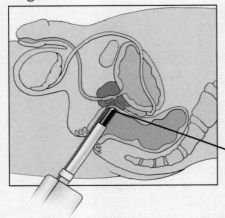

Cancer is detected following a test or procedure for another condition

T1a Cancerous tissue is found in 5% or less of the removed tissue

T1b Cancerous tissue is found in more than 5% of the removed tissue

T1c Cancer is detected from a needle biopsy

Stage II

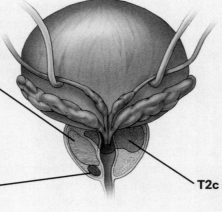

T2b Cancer occupies more than half of one lobe of the prostate

T2a Cancer is confined to half or less of one lobe of the prostate

T2c Cancer is found in both lobes of the prostate

Stage III

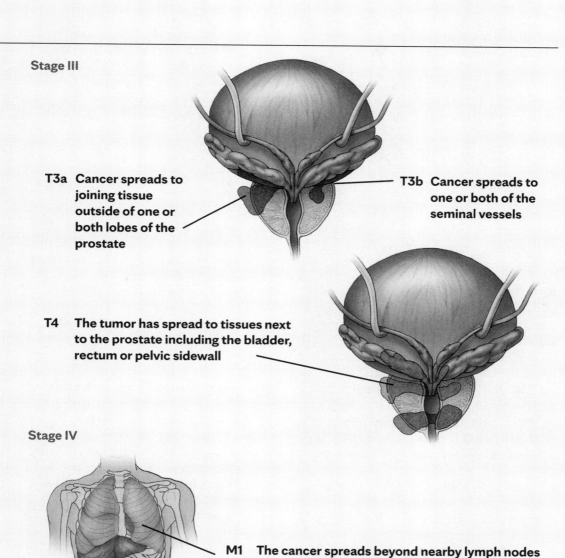

T3a   Cancer spreads to joining tissue outside of one or both lobes of the prostate

T3b   Cancer spreads to one or both of the seminal vessels

T4   The tumor has spread to tissues next to the prostate including the bladder, rectum or pelvic sidewall

Stage IV

M1   The cancer spreads beyond nearby lymph nodes
M1a   To distant lymph nodes
M1b   To the bones
M1c   To other organs, such as lungs, liver or brain

N1, N2, N3   Cancer spreads to nearby lymph nodes

This group is further divided into favorable and unfavorable categories. "Unfavorable intermediate risk" may be given when Gleason score is 7 with a PSA of 10 or greater, Gleason score is 4 + 3 = 7, or more than 50% of your biopsy samples show cancer.

High-risk group

This category equates to a PSA higher than 20 or Gleason score between 8 and 10 or cancer stage at or above T2c.

WHAT'S NEXT?

The decision tree on pages 114-115 helps summarize the path to diagnosis of prostate cancer. Suspicion that cancer has developed — often following an elevated PSA reading or abnormal digital rectal exam during a regular checkup — may lead to an MRI and potentially a biopsy to better determine whether prostate cancer is present.

If cancer cells are found in your biopsy samples, the cells are then studied for their level of aggressiveness and likelihood of spreading outside the prostate (grading). Further testing, including imaging tests, helps determine how far the cancer may have spread (staging).

This knowledge brings you to a critical juncture for deciding how to treat prostate cancer — has the cancer been caught while it remains confined to the prostate (localized), or has it spread to other parts of your body (metastasized)?

Treatment for prostate cancer is different depending on which path you take. Chapters 7 and 8 provide detailed descriptions of therapies to treat prostate cancer and can help guide the decisions that you'll need to make with your doctor.

Surviving prostate cancer

The survival rate for prostate cancer has improved considerably over the past 25 years. According to the American Cancer Society, the death rate for prostate cancer dropped by about 50% between the mid-1990s and mid-2010s. As of 2019 data — the latest available — there were approximately 19 deaths per 100,000 individuals (see the chart on the opposite page).

In the mid-1980s, the 5-year survival rate for adult males with prostate cancer was 76%. Today, the 5-year survival for all stages of prostate cancer combined is almost 100%. Additionally, about 99% of adult males with prostate cancer live at least 10 years past diagnosis. Black men continue to have lower survival rates overall than do white men.

It's hoped that survival figures will continue to improve as efforts are made to try to identify the cancer sooner — in its early stages. For cancer that's diagnosed early and that remains confined to the prostate gland, the survival rate is almost 100%. Doctors also believe that the availability of new treatments for advanced cancer will lead to better survival rates.

CANCER DEATH RATES* BY SITE IN U.S. MALES, 1975-2019

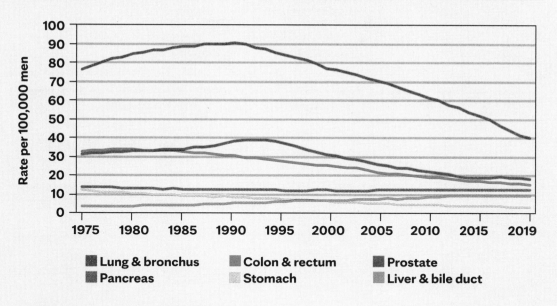

Lung & bronchus   Colon & rectum   Prostate
Pancreas   Stomach   Liver & bile duct

*Per 100,000, age adjusted to the 2000 U.S. standard population.

Based on data from SEER Cancer Statistics Review 1975-2019, National Cancer Institute, 2022.

ANSWERS TO YOUR QUESTIONS

What are tumor markers?

These are substances made from cancerous cells found in your blood. They are also known as biomarkers. When these markers exist in elevated levels, they may indicate the presence of cancer. During treatment and follow-up visits, your blood may be routinely checked for elevated tumor markers. PSA is a tumor marker for prostate cancer.

I have an elevated PSA. Should I have a prostate biopsy?

Remember, elevated PSA levels do not necessarily mean the presence of prostate cancer. Other reasons for high levels of PSA include noncancerous enlargement of the prostate and infections such as prostatitis. PSA levels may rise due to other causes as well, such as recent ejaculation or vigorous exercise involving stimulation of the area between the scrotum and anus (perineum), including bike riding. Of course, elevation in PSA could represent prostate cancer, so it's important to get it checked out.

Whether to get a biopsy is a highly individual decision. As mentioned earlier

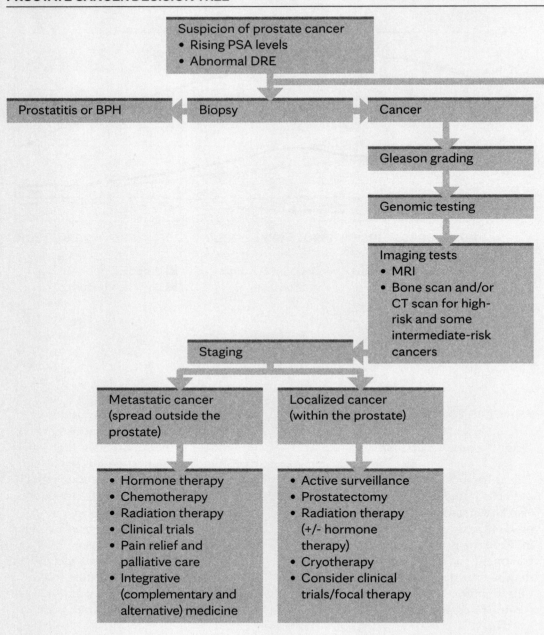

Suspicion of prostate cancer
- Rising PSA levels
- Abnormal DRE

Prostatitis or BPH

Biopsy

Cancer

Gleason grading

Genomic testing

Imaging tests
- MRI
- Bone scan and/or CT scan for high-risk and some intermediate-risk cancers

Staging

Metastatic cancer (spread outside the prostate)

Localized cancer (within the prostate)

- Hormone therapy
- Chemotherapy
- Radiation therapy
- Clinical trials
- Pain relief and palliative care
- Integrative (complementary and alternative) medicine

- Active surveillance
- Prostatectomy
- Radiation therapy (+/- hormone therapy)
- Cryotherapy
- Consider clinical trials/focal therapy

+/- MRI of prostate

- No lesions
- No continued clinical suspicion of prostate cancer (PI-RADS score of 1, 2)

No lesions but continued suspicion of prostate cancer based on PSA, DRE

Positive biopsy (PI-RADS score of 3, 4, 5)

May consider PSA monitoring

Systematic biopsy

Targeted + systematic biopsy

in this chapter, MRI has become increasingly important in helping identify men who may benefit most from a biopsy. If an MRI isn't performed or comes back negative, other testing may be used. For example, PSA density testing can be used to assess the size of the prostate and whether the amount of PSA circulating in the blood is reasonable for the size of a man's prostate. Higher PSA than expected could be a sign of prostate cancer and a biopsy may be recommended. Some men may opt for a biopsy even if PSA density is low.

Additional testing that can help you decide whether to undergo a biopsy includes 4K score, the prostate healthy index (PHI) test, and others. (See pages 30-32 for more on testing options.)

Is a biopsy the only way I can be sure I have prostate cancer?

Yes. Other tests, such as a digital rectal exam, PSA test and an MRI of the prostate, can suggest a strong possibility of prostate cancer. But a biopsy is the only way to be certain that cancer is present.

Can a biopsy be wrong?

When tissue samples are taken from a prostate gland, it's possible to miss the cancer. This is called a sampling error. A biopsy result that comes back normal isn't a guarantee that you don't have cancer. Sampling errors, however, are uncommon.

Can a biopsy loosen cancer cells, allowing them to spread?

No evidence suggests that this can happen. Cancer cells not removed in a biopsy stay within the tumor where they have been growing.

Why do I need to stop taking aspirin before a prostate biopsy?

Aspirin and certain other pain medications thin your blood and can increase your risk of bleeding. Discontinuing these medications for a short period before and after a biopsy will reduce your chances of serious bleeding from the procedure. The same is true for prescription blood thinners taken to reduce clotting, such as warfarin (Coumadin).

Is it possible for a biopsy to cause permanent impotence?

No. Impotence that follows a biopsy is probably due to stress that often accompanies a cancer diagnosis and treatment. In some cases, it may result from temporary inflammation.

I've been diagnosed with prostate cancer. Do I need a PET scan?

PET scans have primarily been used in situations when there's concern about a cancer recurrence after initial treatment — for example, a rising PSA level following radiation or surgery. There are several types of PET scans (see pages 45-47), including the PSMA PET scan.

In general, a PET scan isn't used on initial diagnosis to evaluate an elevated PSA or help in the selection of treatment. However, in men diagnosed with higher-risk prostate cancers where it's suspected the cancer may have spread outside the prostate gland, a PSMA PET scan may be used to get a better look at lymph nodes and organs to see if the cancer has traveled beyond the gland. This can help in deciding on the best option to treat the cancer.

Can I pass cancer on to my partner during sexual intercourse?

No. Cancer cells won't escape from your body through intercourse. Even if they could, they wouldn't be able to grow inside another person because they're genetically coded for your body.

7

Treating prostate cancer

Learning that you have cancer can produce fear, anxiety and sometimes panic. You may feel as if you need to make an immediate decision and begin treating your condition right away. But because prostate cancer is often a slow-growing cancer, there may be no need to rush to a decision regarding treatment.

Give yourself time to sort through your emotions, set priorities and learn about the disease. Develop a strong relationship with your primary physician and the medical team that will be working with you. You'll need to trust their expertise and advice as you consider your treatment options.

If you want additional information, visit the patient education library at your local medical center, if they have one. You can also check out well-respected resources on the internet (see pages 220-221). Write down questions to ask your doctor before the two of you decide on a treatment plan.

You may find it helpful to take a family member or friend with you when you meet with your medical team. There will likely be a lot of new information and unfamiliar medical terminology to sift through, and your emotions might be running high. Your companion can listen, take notes and help you recall the discussion afterward, including what issues still need to be resolved.

TAKING STOCK

There's more than one way to treat prostate cancer. And there's no one best treatment for everybody. Treatment of prostate cancer should be personalized to the circumstances, needs and values of the individual.

In fact, as you evaluate the pros and cons of various therapies, you may find that several treatment options may be available to you. Some men benefit most from a combination of two or more therapies. You may need some time to consider the possibilities.

Which treatment you and your doctor choose will depend on several factors. These include how fast your cancer is growing and how much it has spread, as well as your age, overall health and life expectancy. In addition, you'll need to consider how much the benefits, risks and potential side effects of each treatment may affect you.

ACTIVE SURVEILLANCE

Tests can now help detect prostate cancer at an early stage. Because of this, many men have a greater number of treatment options to consider.

One of these options is to forgo immediate treatment and monitor your condition for signs and symptoms that the cancer is progressing. This is called active surveillance.

Active surveillance is typically reserved for prostate cancer that has a low risk of spreading outside the prostate gland, such as a Gleason score of 6 and a PSA level of less than 10 nanograms per

milliliter (ng/mL). Some men who are a Gleason 3 + 4 may also be candidates for this approach (see page 103 for more about Gleason scoring). Active surveillance may be an option for men with low cancer volume, low PSA density and low risk on genomic testing. It also may be considered in individuals who are unhealthy or have a limited life expectancy.

With active surveillance, there's no medication, radiation or surgery. Instead, you and your doctor keep a close watch on the cancer with regular PSA tests, which are performed about every 6 months. You also may need periodic imaging tests, such as magnetic resonance imaging (MRI), and biopsies. The goal is to catch the disease at the earliest stages of progression — usually to a higher grade — and treat it at that time, when there's still a very good chance for a cure.

If you're fairly young — in your 40s or 50s — and healthy at the time of diagnosis, active surveillance may be an option. However, keep in mind that because of your age, you're more likely to eventually need treatment, as the cancer will have many years to develop. Even with a small, slow-growing tumor, cancer cells may eventually spread so extensively that a cure becomes difficult or impossible.

Among some men, genomic testing of biopsy tissue can help decide who's a good candidate for active surveillance. This testing allows doctors to better predict which cancers might be aggressive. (See page 105 for more about genomic testing.)

ACTIVE SURVEILLANCE VERSUS WATCHFUL WAITING

Sometimes active surveillance is confused with watchful waiting. Watchful waiting is often used for individuals who are too unhealthy to undergo treatment or have a limited life expectancy. Watchful waiting refers to waiting to treat the cancer until symptoms develop, generally when the cancer spreads outside the prostate gland, usually to bone.

Rather than focusing on curing the cancer, treatment is aimed at minimizing symptoms — for example, back pain if prostate cancer has spread to the bones of the back. In the majority of cases of watchful waiting, hormone therapy is the most common treatment for control of symptoms (see page 146).

Are you a candidate?

You may be considered a candidate for active surveillance if:
- The cancer is slow growing and confined to the prostate (typically a Gleason 6 score).
- You're willing to take the risk that you might miss the window of opportunity for a cure.

Benefits

The benefits of active surveillance include:
- You avoid side effects, such as erectile dysfunction or incontinence, associated with other treatments.
- You buy time to consider your treatment options — it can take several years for a tiny tumor to double in size. Research suggests that between 50% and 68% of candidates for active surveillance safely avoid treatment for at least 10 years.
- You can choose to treat your cancer at a later date if the risk level increases.

Risks

Two key risks are associated with active surveillance:
- The cancer may grow while you wait. Although uncommon, a slow-growing cancer may become a fast-growing one. In such cases, the cancer may require more extensive treatment that results in more severe side effects than if it had been treated earlier.
- You may become what's called the walking worried — anxious about your health and preoccupied with test results. Although more aggressive treatment has its risks, it may reduce the fear that you're gambling with your life.

PROSTATE CANCER SURGERY

Surgical removal of the entire prostate gland is an effective means of treating cancer that's confined to the gland. This type of surgery is called radical prostatectomy.

A majority of men in their 40s and 50s, and many in their 60s, choose radical prostatectomy. Men in their 70s may prefer other options, such as radiation therapy, over surgery. And men in their 80s and beyond tend to choose no treatment at all.

New procedures and technology developed during the past two decades have considerably changed how this type of surgery is performed. Surgeons use special techniques to completely remove the prostate and nearby lymph nodes while producing fewer complications and side effects.

Newer techniques aim to spare muscles and nerves close to the prostate gland that control urination and sexual function. In the past, muscles and nerves may have been permanently damaged or severed. Improved techniques also are resulting in less bleeding and less need for a transfusion, as well as improving safety and recovery time.

Radical prostatectomy is usually performed under general anesthesia. Historically, two primary open surgical approaches were used: retropubic and perineal. The perineal approach, which involves making an incision between the anus and scrotum, is rarely performed anymore because of significant disadvantages. They include an inability to access and remove lymph nodes for testing, as well as problems with sparing nerve bundles.

Open (retropubic) surgery

With retropubic surgery, the prostate gland is removed through an incision in the lower abdomen. The incision typically runs between the navel and the pubic bone, a couple of inches above the base of the penis. (See the illustration on page 15 as a guide to pelvic anatomy.)

This is the most common form of open prostate removal for two reasons. First, a surgeon can remove pelvic lymph nodes through the same incision. Second, the procedure gives the surgeon better access to the gland, making it easier to spare the muscles and nerves that help control bladder function and penile erections.

Removing the prostate requires detaching the organ from the bottom of the bladder. In addition, the urethra is severed below the prostate gland but above the external sphincter muscle that helps control urine flow. The vasa deferentia, which carry sperm from the testicles to the urethra, also must be cut. The seminal vesicles, which are potential sites for cancer spread, are removed along with the prostate gland.

Once the prostate is removed, the surgeon reattaches your urethra to your bladder. This reconnection allows you to urinate normally, although it may take several days to a few weeks — or in some cases, months — for your body to heal sufficiently and for you to regain full bladder control.

Open surgery typically requires 1 to 2 days in the hospital, then 3 to 5 weeks of additional recovery at home. A catheter is inserted into your bladder to drain urine while tissues heal. You'll need the catheter for about 1 to 2 weeks to give your urinary tract time to heal.

Robotic surgery

Robot-assisted laparoscopic radical prostatectomy (RALRP) is a minimally invasive surgical approach for prostate cancer. Robotic surgery is performed under general anesthesia. Five or six tiny incisions are made in the abdomen through which a surgeon inserts special instruments, including a long, slender tube that contains a camera (laparoscope). The laparoscope provides the surgeon with a magnified view of the surgical area.

All instruments are attached to a mechanical device that's controlled by the surgeon, who guides the instruments while seated at a console equipped with a highly specialized monitor. Robotic techniques provide precision and accuracy in removing the prostate gland and sparing the nerves around it.

Robotic surgery is now the most common procedure for removing the prostate gland after a diagnosis of prostate cancer. More than 90% of all prostatectomies in the United States are done with robotic assistance. To get the best outcomes and minimize side effects, it's important to find a surgeon experienced in robotic surgery and an institution with extensive

LYMPH NODE REMOVAL

During a prostatectomy, a surgeon may remove the lymph nodes near the prostate gland and send tissue samples to a pathologist to check for cancer spread. Enlarged or suspect lymph nodes can be evaluated during surgery in a process called frozen section to determine if cancer is present. Results are often known within 15 to 30 minutes of removal.

Removal of adjacent lymph nodes helps a surgeon better understand the extent of the cancer — specifically, whether it's spread beyond the prostate or is still confined to the gland. This knowledge also helps determine prognosis and guides any additional treatment that may be needed, such as radiation or hormone therapy.

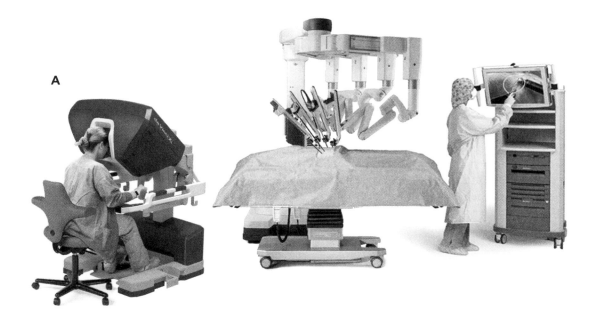

Robot-assisted surgery While performing robot-assisted surgery, the surgeon sits at a computer console that's several feet away from the operating table (A). The robotic device has several mechanical arms equipped with specially designed instruments. Each mechanical arm features a flexible "wrist" that's capable of greater range of movement than the human wrist. The surgeon uses hand controls on the computer console to manipulate the robotic instruments (B). The tiny tools move in real time with the surgeon's hand movements (C).

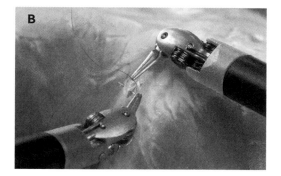

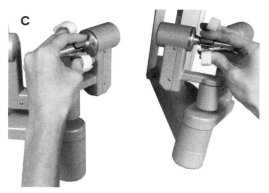

experience in caring for men who've undergone a robotic prostatectomy. An experienced surgeon can often complete the operation in about 2 to 3 hours and the surgeon performs more than 50 prostatectomies a year.

Robotic surgery generally provides greater precision and produces less bleeding, has a faster recovery time and usually requires shorter hospital stays (often a day) than conventional open surgery. It also may cause less pain.

Are you a candidate?

You may be a candidate for radical prostatectomy if:
- Your prostate cancer hasn't spread to bone or lymph nodes. Some men whose cancer has spread to lymph nodes may be candidates.
- You're healthy enough to withstand the surgery.

Benefits

For cancer that's confined to the prostate gland, surgery is a very effective treatment option. If the cancer hasn't spread to organs and tissue in other parts of your body, it's very possible to remove all the cancer cells and cure your disease.

A benefit of surgery is that it generally avoids the need for treatment that shuts off testosterone in the body, known as androgen-deprivation therapy, or hormone therapy. Hormone therapy generally isn't necessary prior to surgery. Surgery avoids side effects associated with hormone therapy, such as hot flashes, fatigue, loss of muscle mass, loss of sex drive and osteoporosis.

Risks

All major surgery carries some risk, including a low risk of death, which increases with age. Other risks include the following.
- You may experience erectile dysfunction after the procedure. This depends on your age, the skill of your surgeon and the quality of your erections before surgery. If you have good erectile function before surgery and nerves are spared, your chances of being able to have erections again improve.
- You may experience urinary incontinence. This is usually temporary, with the vast majority of men recovering within six months of surgery. After the catheter is removed, nearly all men have some bladder control problems for a few weeks. During this time, conservative measures such as pads are used to manage the incontinence. Pelvic floor muscle training also may be used to help speed recovery of urinary control.
- There's a small risk of damage to your lower intestine or rectum. Additional surgery may be necessary to repair this damage.

More on erectile dysfunction

Depending on where the cancer is located, your surgeon will try to save the

Before leaving the hospital, you'll receive instructions from your health care team about caring for yourself during your recovery. These instructions will likely address the following:

Catheter use. After surgery you'll need to wear a urinary catheter to allow for healing of the juncture where the urethra was reattached to your bladder. Follow the instructions you're given carefully — they're designed to help prevent infection and blockage of urine. Drinking fluids is especially important in the 7 to 10 days you have the catheter in place. This helps to keep urine flowing freely and reduces the chance of blockage.

When your catheter is removed, you may experience some leakage of urine. That's because it takes time for the swelling to resolve and for the pelvic muscles to regain their strength. You may need to wear protective underwear for several days, and an absorbent pad after that. Daily muscle strengthening exercises (Kegels) may be helpful. They can help reduce or eliminate your incontinence but be patient. It can take a few months to notice the effects.

Constipation. To help avoid constipation, eat plenty of fruits and vegetables and avoid red meat and pork for a couple of weeks. Oral stool softeners also can help treat post-surgery constipation. It's important not to have enemas or rectal examinations for a few months after surgery. (See Chapter 9 for more on constipation.)

Medications. Make a list on a sheet of paper all of the medications you need to take daily. Include check-off spaces for doses and times.

Exercise. Don't become a couch potato during your recovery. Staying active is important, and walking is an excellent form of exercise. Movement helps prevent the development of blood clots in your legs, which can be life-threatening. See your doctor if you develop redness or tenderness in the area of a leg vein. Moving around also helps strengthen the pelvic floor muscles, which can help you regain urine control. (See Chapter 9 for more on pelvic floor muscles.)

Hygiene. Over time, incontinence can cause a rash near the tip of the penis. This could be a yeast infection called balanitis. Your doctor can prescribe an antifungal cream. Wash your penis with soap and water daily and dry it thoroughly before applying the cream. Antifungal medication can help clear up the infection and prevent a recurrence.

neurovascular bundles attached to each side of the prostate gland. These nerves control your ability to have an erection. Often, one or both of the bundles can be spared.

Men in their 40s and 50s who undergo this procedure are more likely to retain their ability to have an erection than are older men. For some older men — especially those who aren't sexually active — even spared nerves won't survive the shock of surgery and recovery of erectile function is less likely.

If even one nerve bundle is spared after the procedure, it's still possible for you to have erections. If neither nerve bundle can be spared, spontaneous erections are unlikely without treatment (see Chapter 9). Even if your ability to have erections is lost, you can still have a normal sex drive (libido), your sensation is unchanged, and you can still experience orgasms.

Regardless of the outcome, no fluid will be produced with an orgasm after surgery. That's because the structures that make and transport semen — the prostate gland, seminal vesicles and vasa deferentia — have been either removed or disconnected. The fact that you have dry orgasms has no effect on sensation, but it does mean that you won't be able to father children without medical help.

RADIATION THERAPY

Radiation is used to treat many different types of cancer, and it's been a treatment for prostate cancer for nearly a century. High-powered X-rays or other types of radiation interfere with the ability of cancer cells to reproduce. Cancer cells are generally more susceptible to radiation's harmful effects than are normal cells. This means it's possible to selectively destroy cancer cells while minimizing damage to normal tissue.

Radiation therapy may be used for all stages of prostate cancer. If the cancer has spread, radiation may be used to help slow progression of the disease, delay the need for changes in a treatment and improve quality of life, even when a cure isn't possible.

External beam radiotherapy

When radiation is delivered from a device outside the body, it's called external beam radiotherapy (EBRT). The radiation is most commonly generated by a machine called a linear accelerator that can target a concentrated beam directly to the prostate gland.

Because the radiation can also damage healthy tissue next to the prostate, including the bladder and rectum, precisely locating the beam is necessary to reduce negative side effects.

Intensity-modulated radiation therapy (IMRT)

This form of external beam radiotherapy uses high-powered X-rays to kill cancer cells. For better accuracy, IMRT uses

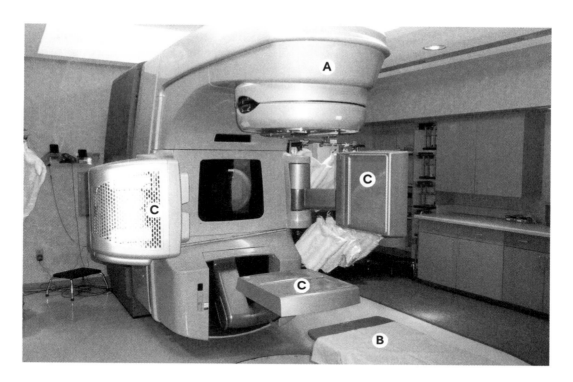

External beam radiotherapy Radiation is delivered from a large, movable gantry (A) to an individual lying on the treatment table (B), which will be positioned below the gantry. Imaging devices (C) permit the radiologist to closely monitor the procedure.

custom-made body supports prepared specifically for each person and for each treatment angle. These supports maintain the body in the same position from one visit to the next.

The body supports help reduce the size of the area receiving a full dose of radiation, significantly limiting damage to adjacent tissue and reducing side effects. Broader areas may be treated with X-rays if there's concern the cancer has spread beyond the prostate. Long-term outcomes for most men receiving IMRT are generally positive.

A first step in the procedure is to map the precise areas of your body that need to receive radiation. A radiation oncology specialist uses computerized tomography (CT) to determine the exact locations of the prostate gland and surrounding organs and to plan radiation doses. Computer software allows the specialist to rotate a 3D image to find the best angles to fire the beam and deliver strong doses of radiation.

Treatments are generally given on an outpatient basis every 1 to 2 days for approximately 2 to 7 weeks, based on your individual characteristics and cancer stage. Each treatment takes about 15 minutes, although most of this is preparation time. Radiation is received for only a few minutes. Anesthesia isn't needed because there's no sensation of pain.

For the actual procedure, you lie motionless on a treatment table while the linear accelerator moves about you, targeting the cancer. To ensure the beams always hit the mark, body supports hold you in the same position for each session. Custom-designed shields are positioned to cover parts of your body such as the intestines, anus and urethra, protecting them from scattered rays. This precau-

tion allows the technician to apply higher doses of radiation than would otherwise be possible.

Other measures may be taken to improve accuracy. You may be asked to arrive with a full bladder, which helps hold your prostate in the same position and keeps sensitive tissue further away from the radiation beam. Ink marks or small tattoos placed on your skin can serve as visual targeting guides.

A common method uses small metallic markers to precisely locate the prostate before each treatment. These markers are inserted into the prostate using a method

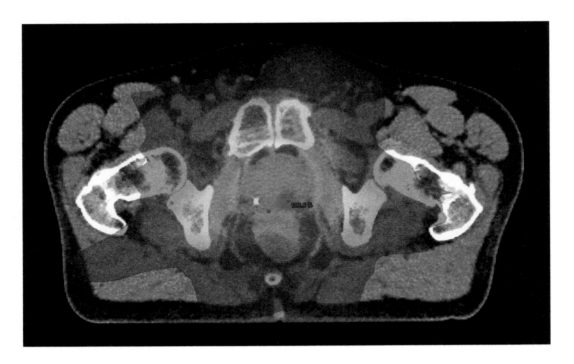

IMRT dosage An axial CT image taken after IMRT shows the radiation area (green shading) to treat cancer of the prostate gland (red shading).

similar to that used to biopsy tissue before IMRT begins. Once implanted, imaging equipment uses the markers to determine the best position of the beam for maximum effect and the least damage to surrounding tissue.

X-ray imaging and a type of CT scan built into the linear accelerator, known as a cone-beam CT, are frequently used to image internal organs and the cancerous region to adjust the radiation beams during each treatment. This ensures that the appropriate regions are targeted.

Proton beam

This external beam method uses the positively charged parts of an atom (protons) instead of X-rays to destroy the cancer. Unlike conventional X-rays, protons deposit most of their energy only when they reach their target. This allows more of the radiation dose to be delivered directly to the target, while decreasing some of the dose to nearby organs, such as the rectum and bladder.

Advances continue to be made in the field of proton therapy. Similar to IMRT, intensity-modulated proton therapy (IMPT) uses a spot-scanning method. This allows better conformity of the radiation dose to the target, further sparing the healthy organs nearby.

Proton beam therapy is still being investigated, but it's thought the treatment can be at least as effective as conventional external beam radiotherapy in treating prostate cancer, while reducing the risk of short- and long-term side effects of radiotherapy. There have been an increasing number of studies demonstrating the safety and effectiveness of proton therapy for the treatment of prostate cancer in recent years. Proton therapy may be used alone or in combination with conventional external beam radiotherapy.

Combination treatment

External beam radiotherapy may be used in conjunction with hormone therapy (see Chapter 8). Studies have shown that in men with high-risk prostate cancer and certain forms of intermediate-risk prostate cancer, survival improves if they have received both external beam radiation and hormone therapy, compared with either treatment alone.

Hormone therapy may last for a few months to 2 years or more — the duration depends on the cancer. External beam radiation may proceed hormone therapy, but it typically overlaps it for a period.

External beam radiotherapy also may be performed shortly after you've had cancer surgery, even if there's no sign of remaining cancer. This approach may be recommended when the pathology report indicates it's likely that the cancer will recur. Use of radiation in this manner is called adjuvant radiotherapy.

Recurrent cancer

External beam radiation is often used when there's an indication that the cancer has recurred — usually signaled by a rising PSA level. This is known as salvage radiotherapy. Early salvage radiotherapy is as effective as adjuvant radiotherapy in controlling local recurrence and reducing the risk of distant cancer spread and prostate cancer-related death.

Salvage radiotherapy is often combined with hormone therapy. The target area for this type of treatment may be limited to where the prostate gland used to be (prostatic bed) or it may be extended to cover both the prostatic bed and the pelvic lymph node region.

There's some debate regarding which treatment — adjuvant radiotherapy or salvage radiation therapy — is more effective after surgery. Emerging studies seem to indicate that salvage radiation treatment may be as effective as adjuvant radiation, particularly when applied in the early stages of recurrence. For more on cancer recurrence, see Chapter 8.

Radioactive seed implants

Another method of delivering radiation to cancer cells in the prostate is called brachytherapy. Rather than using an external device, this procedure delivers radiation directly to the gland, providing a higher dose of radiation than with external beams and potentially causing less damage to surrounding tissues.

Brachytherapy may be used alone or in combination with hormone therapy or external beam radiotherapy. There are two main methods used in the treatment of prostate cancer: permanent seed implant and temporary seed implant.

Permanent seed implant

This method implants low-dose-rate radioactive seeds into the prostate gland, which emit radiation over several weeks or months. The tiny seeds may contain one of several radioactive substances, called isotopes. The most commonly used low-energy isotopes for this purpose are iodine 125 and palladium 103.

Hollow needles inject the radioactive seeds in and around the gland. The needles pass through the skin of your perineum — the area between your scrotum and anus — to reach the gland. An ultrasound probe inserted into your rectum guides the placement of the seeds. A template attached to the probe and held up against your perineum helps steady the loaded needles.

With this method, the seeds:
- Usually remain in place permanently, even after they stop emitting radiation.
- Emit radiation that generally extends only a few millimeters beyond their location and doesn't escape the prostate area.
- Lose nearly all radiation within a year.

Between 50 and 120 seeds may be inserted into the gland. The total number depends on the size of your prostate and other factors. The procedure lasts about 1 to 2 hours and is done on an outpatient basis using either general anesthesia or a spinal block, which numbs the lower body.

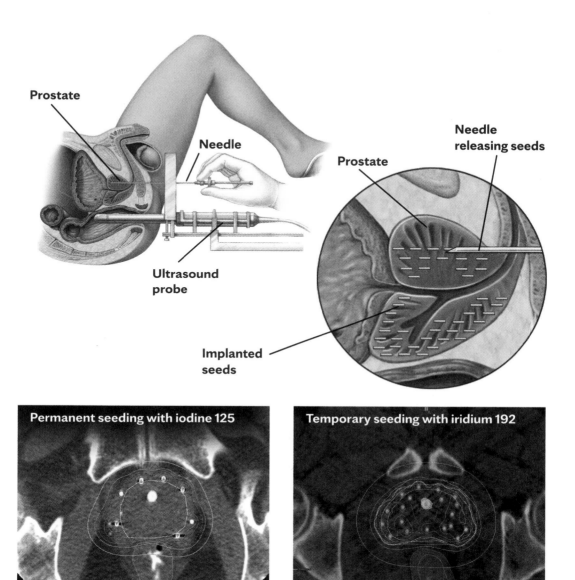

Prostate

Needle

Ultrasound probe

Prostate

Needle releasing seeds

Implanted seeds

Permanent seeding with iodine 125

Temporary seeding with iridium 192

Permanent and temporary seed implantation In the CT image on the left, each white dot (except the center one) indicates a seed of iodine 125 that has been permanently implanted in the prostate. The image on the right represents high-dose-rate therapy. Each white dot is a needle through which a source of iridium 192 will be placed temporarily in the prostate. Colored lines in both images represent a specially calculated radiation dose.

Temporary seed implant

This method, known as high-dose-rate (HDR) brachytherapy, also places a radioactive source directly into your prostate. However, the source doesn't remain in your body.

For the procedure, small hollow needles are placed into the prostate. A computer-controlled machine then pushes a high-dose-rate radioactive source (iridium 192) into each needle to deliver a dose of radiation to the prostate.

With use of a computer, your doctor can control the radiation dose to the prostate and nearby organs. This enables your doctor to deliver a targeted radiation dose to your prostate, while minimizing radiation to the rectum and bladder. The ability to modify the radiation dose after the needles are placed is one of the main advantages of high-dose-rate brachytherapy over permanent seed implants. A disadvantage of the procedure is that it may require more treatments than with a permanent seed procedure.

Once the procedure is completed, the needles are removed, and no radioactive seeds are left in your prostate gland. High-dose-rate brachytherapy may be performed in one procedure, or in two or more procedures done 1 to 4 weeks apart.

Similar to permanent seed implant, the therapy can be used alone or in combination with external beam radiotherapy. A combination treatment is usually recommended for men with high-risk prostate cancer. Hormone therapy also may be combined with high-dose-rate brachytherapy in certain situations.

---

10 QUESTIONS TO ASK YOUR DOCTOR

To better understand your best treatment options, ask these 10 questions at the next visit to your doctor:
1. What options are available?
2. How fast will the cancer grow if left untreated?
3. Can the cancer be cured with treatment? If so, what are the chances?
4. Which treatment would you recommend and why?
5. How many times have you performed this procedure?
6. How soon before we know if the treatment has worked?
7. What are the risks of experiencing long-term side effects, such as erectile dysfunction or incontinence?
8. How soon is it possible to return to work?
9. Will any activities have to be restricted?
10. If a particular treatment doesn't work, are there other options?

High-dose-rate brachytherapy is considered safe and effective. Researchers continue to examine various treatment regimens. The procedure is generally easier to perform on small or moderate-size prostates, but men with larger prostates also may be considered for the treatment. Some men with very large prostates or a narrow pelvis may undergo hormone therapy to shrink the prostate.

Are you a candidate?

You may be a candidate for radiation therapy if:
- Your cancer can't be cured by surgery alone — often because it has spread outside the prostate.
- You don't want surgery.
- You're not a candidate for surgery for reasons such as previous abdominal or pelvic surgeries and other health conditions that make surgery less safe.
- You expect to live longer than your cancer would allow you to live.

Benefits

External beam radiotherapy and brachytherapy are both effective treatments for prostate cancer and can cure your disease. Additional benefits include:
- Both forms of radiation therapy are generally done on an outpatient basis. With brachytherapy, you may spend one night in the hospital.
- EBRT is a noninvasive treatment that doesn't involve general anesthesia.
- Recovery is generally less difficult and takes less time compared to surgery.

Risks

Radiation side effects can start immediately; however, they're usually delayed. Risks include the following:
- Radiation therapy may affect sexual function by damaging nerves that control erections and arteries that carry blood to the penis. Most men don't have problems with erections at the beginning of therapy, but eventually many experience them. Your age and the amount of radiation you receive affect your risk.
- It may produce urinary problems. The most common complaints are more frequent and urgent needs to urinate or a burning sensation while urinating. These problems tend to be temporary and gradually improve a few weeks after treatment. In some cases, symptoms recur several years later. Symptoms tend to be worse and last longer with brachytherapy than with external beam radiation.
- Some men who undergo external beam radiation experience colorectal problems, including increased bowel movements, rectal bleeding, a burning sensation around the anus and urgency to have a bowel movement. These issues generally subside when the treatments cease, but for some men the problems may persist or recur after several years as a delayed side effect. Fortunately, with recent advances in the targeting of radiation, these side effects are less common. With seed implantation, rectal problems are uncommon.

With permanent seed implants, the amount of radiation detectable at the skin's surface after implantation is very small. While the Nuclear Regulatory Commission states that no specific precautions are required, it may be appropriate to avoid prolonged close contact (less than a foot) with small children or pregnant women. Within a year, all radiation inside the pellets is generally exhausted. Use of temporary implants doesn't require special precautions because no radiation remains in your body after treatment is completed.

FOCAL THERAPY

As treatments and techniques evolve in prostate cancer care, there's been increasing interest in limiting treatment-related side effects and improving quality of life. One way of accomplishing this is to restrict how much of the prostate gland is treated, an approach called focal therapy. With focal therapy, a small portion (quadrant) or half of the prostate gland is treated while sparing noninvolved tissue.

Similar approaches have been used in other cancers. For example, kidney cancers are commonly treated by removing or destroying only the tumor while leaving the rest of the kidney intact and functioning. Improvements in prostate imaging and biopsy techniques make it easier to better identify the location of the cancer within the prostate and identify individuals who may be candidates for focal therapy.

Ideal candidates have intermediate-risk prostate cancer that's localized to a single area of the prostate. Some men who have more than one area of cancer within the gland may still be candidates, provided other areas of cancer are low grade (Gleason 6) and low volume.

The tumor that's targeted is referred to as the index lesion. In glands that have more than one tumor, the index lesion is generally the largest tumor with the highest grade. It's believed that the index lesion drives the behavior of the prostate cancer and that treating it alone with focal therapy may lead to good overall cancer control with fewer side effects.

Focal therapy generally uses extremely high or extremely low temperatures to destroy very specific areas of tissue (ablation). This allows for precise destruction of cancerous tissue while avoiding structures important for normal sexual and urinary function.

Focal therapy is a relatively new treatment option that has less robust evidence compared with conventional treatments. This approach is still considered investigational, but it's an area of great interest and research. No clinical guidelines currently recommend it for treatment of prostate cancer, but focal therapy is increasingly available.

Focal therapy outcomes may be influenced by the location of the tumor within the prostate. The tumor being located closer to the rectum, urethra or a nerve bundle can make treatment more difficult. In some cases, focal therapy may not be curative and additional treatment for prostate cancer may be necessary.

Following focal therapy, regular follow-up is important for identifying any recurrence or new cancer. Patients require regular PSA testing, intermittent MRIs, and usually additional prostate biopsies as part of the follow-up program. In general, follow-up is more frequent compared with conventional treatments like surgery or radiation therapy.

While the data is still limited, the short- and intermediate-term outcomes of focal therapy are promising. At 5 years, approximately 80% of focal therapy candidates have been able to avoid additional treatment, such as surgery or radiation. Men who experience residual or recurrent cancer after focal therapy may be retreated with additional focal therapy or they may undergo surgery or radiation therapy.

Focal cryoablation

One form of focal therapy used in the treatment of prostate cancer uses cryoablation, also known as cryotherapy. It involves freezing prostate tissue to kill the cancer cells. The prostate tissue dies in place and is reabsorbed by the body.

The procedure involves inserting several thin metal probes (cryoneedles), each about 6 inches (15 centimeters) long, through the perineum and into the portion of the prostate gland that contains the tumor. A doctor uses either an ultrasound probe that's inserted into the rectum or MRI to help position the needles.

Once the needles are in place, argon gas is circulated through them, which plunges their temperature enough to freeze the tissue around them. As tissue near the needles freezes, cancerous cells rupture and die. During the freezing process, a warming catheter, which contains warm saline, is placed into the urethra to protect its tissues from freezing.

After the tissue is frozen, helium gas is then circulated through the needles to thaw the needles and tissue. This freeze-thaw cycle may be repeated two more times to destroy the optimal amount of tissue. Throughout the process, the needle temperatures are controlled with a computer.

The entire procedure takes about 2 to 4 hours. About 60 to 90 minutes of that time is spent performing the freeze-thaw cycles.

Most patients will be able to go home the same day as the procedure. You'll probably be able to return to normal activities in about two weeks. It will take your body about nine months to a year to reabsorb the destroyed tissues.

Sometimes cryoablation is performed on the entire prostate (whole-gland cryotherapy). This approach is generally reserved for men with low- and intermediate-risk prostate cancer who aren't candidates for either radical prostatectomy or radiotherapy due to other health conditions but have a life expectancy of 10 years or longer. The risk of side effects is higher when the whole prostate gland is treated.

Are you a candidate?

You may be a good candidate for focal cryoablation if:
- Your cancer is confined to one spot in the prostate gland.
- You don't want to undergo surgery or radiation therapy.

Benefits

Benefits of focal cryoablation include:
- Lower risk for side effects, including urinary incontinence and erectile dysfunction, compared to surgery or radiation therapy.
- Performed as a minimally invasive outpatient procedure.
- Quicker recovery than surgery.
- Less time commitment than radiation.
- Can potentially be repeated if needed.
- Does not limit future ability to have radiation therapy or surgical treatment.

Risks

With all types of focal therapy, a risk is that the treatment may not kill all cancer cells on the first try and may have to be repeated. Other potential issues include:
- Risk of erectile dysfunction, depending on how close the treatment zone is to the nerve bundles that control erections. This is more common with whole-gland cryotherapy.
- Trouble urinating for several weeks. This is because freezing swells the prostate, which squeezes the urethra. You may also experience urinary infections, pain or burning with urina-

tion, blood in your urine, urinary incontinence and scarring that restricts the flow of urine (urethral stricture). Symptoms may temporarily worsen before they get better.
- Absent or decreased ejaculation.
- Infection or inflammation leading to temporary swelling in the testicles and/ or the tube that stores and carries sperm (epididymo-orchitis).
- Chronic pelvic pain.
- In rare cases, an abnormal connection between the urethra and the rectum or anus (fistula).

Although short-term results of focal therapies look encouraging, long-term survival rates are still unknown.

High-intensity focused ultrasound

High-intensity focused ultrasound (HIFU) treatment uses concentrated ultrasound energy to destroy (ablate) prostate tissue. The procedure is done while an individual is under general anesthesia. A special ultrasound probe is placed in the rectum. This probe is used to both image the prostate gland and deliver treatment. There are no incisions or needles used.

Once the initial positioning and planning steps are complete, treatment is delivered. Each HIFU treatment lasts just a few seconds and destroys an area of tissue that's about the size of a grain of rice. An ablation zone is created by delivering multiple treatments to cover a predefined area of the prostate, based on imaging and biopsy results.

During treatment, the surgeon is given real-time imaging and information that helps assess the success of the ablation. How long the procedure takes depends on the size of the area to be ablated, but in general takes approximately 2 hours.

HIFU is well tolerated and is done as a same-day, outpatient procedure. A catheter is put in during the procedure and is usually left in place for 5 to 7 days afterward to allow for healing. Most men are able to resume normal activities in a day or two.

HIFU has also been used to ablate the entire prostate gland. The risk of side effects is higher when the whole prostate is treated.

TULSA

An alternative type of ultrasound-based ablation is called transurethral ultrasound ablation (TULSA). This procedure uses a special probe placed in the urethra to transmit ultrasound energy into the prostate. The procedure is performed under general anesthesia within an MRI scanner. It can be used for partial or whole prostate treatment. The technology can also be used to treat symptoms of benign prostatic hyperplasia (BPH).

Am I a candidate?

You may be a candidate for HIFU if:
- Your prostate cancer is intermediate-risk and located in only one area of the prostate, preferably in the back.

- Your prostate is small- to moderate-size. Some men with large prostates may still be candidates if the tumor is located on the back of the prostate.
- Your prostate has no major prostate calcifications or large cysts, which can hinder treatment delivery.
- You're in otherwise good health, having no bowel disease or prior significant rectal surgery.

Benefits

Some of the benefits of HIFU include:
- Lower risk for functional side effects, including urinary incontinence and erectile dysfunction, compared to surgery or radiation therapy.
- Minimally invasive outpatient procedure.
- Quicker recovery than surgery.
- Less time commitment compared to radiation.
- Can potentially be repeated if needed.
- Doesn't limit the future ability to have radiation therapy or surgical treatment.

Risks

Focal HIFU may not kill all the cancer on the first try, and it may have to be repeated. Other potential issues include:
- Most men experience some temporary symptoms including urinary urgency, frequency, a slower stream, and burning or discomfort. Side effects can be managed with medications, and symptoms typically improve within a few weeks.
- Urinary incontinence and erectile dysfunction can occur. Rates are

generally lower than with prostate surgery but depend on the specific location being treated. Other side effects include urinary retention, urinary infection, problems ejaculating, urethral stricture and, rarely, a rectal fistula.

Laser ablation therapy

An additional treatment option is called laser interstitial thermal therapy (LITT), also called laser ablation therapy. Laser ablation is a minimally invasive technique that uses laser light to deposit high-energy particles into prostate tissue, causing tissue destruction through rapid heating.

The procedure uses MRI as a guide to move the laser applicators through the perineum into the prostate gland and to monitor treatment. When the applicators are in place, gentle heating is performed to confirm their position. Once in the optimal spot, laser energy is applied to heat the area and destroy cancerous tissue. Once the targeted area is fully destroyed, the application of heat is stopped before it affects other areas. During treatment, a cooling catheter, which circulates cool saline, is placed into the urethra to protect urethral tissue from overheating.

The entire procedure takes about 2 to 4 hours, most of which is used for placement of the applicators. Laser ablation itself takes only about 10 minutes. You may stay in the hospital overnight and should be able to return to normal activities in about a week. The ablated tissue will be slowly reabsorbed by your body over about 9 months to a year.

Are you a candidate?

You may be a good candidate for laser ablation if:
- Your tumor is small and confined to one spot in the prostate.
- You don't want to undergo surgery or radiation therapy.

Benefits

Benefits of laser ablation therapy include:
- Lower risk of side effects, including urinary incontinence and erectile dysfunction, compared to surgery or radiation therapy.
- Minimally invasive outpatient procedure.
- Quicker recovery than surgery.
- Less time commitment compared to radiation.
- Can potentially be repeated if needed.
- Does not limit the future ability to have radiation therapy or surgical treatment.

Risks

Laser therapy doesn't always kill all the cancer on the first try, and the procedure may have to be repeated. There are other potential side effects:
- There's a risk of erectile dysfunction depending on how close the treatment zone is to the nerve bundles that control erections.

- Trouble urinating for several weeks. This is because laser ablation may lead to local swelling within the prostate, which squeezes the urethra.
- Infection.

Although short-term results of laser ablation therapy look encouraging, long-term survival rates are unknown.

Irreversible electroporation

Irreversible electroporation (IRE) uses electricity to damage prostate cancer cells without exposing adjacent tissues to heat.

During the procedure, thin needlelike probes are placed into the prostate gland through the skin in the perineum. Short but strong electrical fields are generated between the probes to create small holes in cancer cells, killing the cells. The procedure is guided by ultrasound and MRI fusion technology to ensure the most accurate treatment.

This outpatient procedure takes approximately 1 to 2 hours and is performed under general anesthesia.

Are you a candidate?

You may be a candidate for IRE if:
- Your cancer is confined to one location in the prostate gland.
- You don't have certain implanted electronic devices.
- You don't want to undergo surgery or radiation therapy.

Benefits

The benefits of IRE include:
- The procedure is generally well tolerated.
- It minimizes potential damage to nearby structures.
- Stress-based urinary incontinence is rare.

Risks

Focal IRE may not kill all the cancer cells on the first try and have to be repeated. Most men notice slight decreases in erections following the procedure. However, men with good erectile function prior to the procedure generally recover normal erections within 12 months. There also may be a reduction in semen volume.

Other potential side effects include:
- Temporary urinary symptoms, such as bleeding.
- Infection.
- Cardiac arrhythmia.
- Muscle injury and injury to nearby structures.
- Blood clots.
- Injury to adjacent structures.
- Risks associated with anesthesia.

EMERGING TREATMENTS

Initial study results suggest that the following therapies may prove to be viable treatment options for men facing early-stage prostate cancer. Further study is needed to better assess how the outcomes of these treatments compare with standard treatments after 5 or more years.

Some of the new treatments under development include the following:

- **Lutetium-177-PSMA-617.** This is a type of radiation therapy that targets prostate-specific membrane antigen (PSMA), which is found in metastatic prostate cancer and is a common indicator for decreased survival. Targeting PSMA has been shown to slow disease progression and improve survival.
- **Photodynamic therapy.** This is another type of focal therapy. It's a two-stage treatment that combines light energy with a drug (photosensitizer) designed to destroy cancerous and precancerous cells after light activation. Photosensitizers are activated by a specific wavelength of light energy, usually from a laser. In research studies, photodynamic therapy has shown promise in treating prostate cancer, while minimizing side effects such as erectile dysfunction and urinary incontinence.

THINGS TO CONSIDER

Selecting a treatment that will work best for you means weighing all the options in relation to your overall health, needs, values and lifestyle. As you make your decision, here are issues to consider and questions to ask yourself and your doctor.

How much time should you take to make your decision?

Consider the aggressiveness of your prostate cancer; is it likely to grow rapidly or slowly? Many prostate cancers are slow-growing and may not require immediate treatment, so there may be no need to rush your decision. Several studies indicate that waiting to treat high-risk prostate cancers within 6 months of the diagnosis generally doesn't change cancer outcomes.

What's the current state of your general health?

Are there other conditions that may affect your health over the next few years? If you're young and relatively healthy, you may want to consider more aggressive treatment options, which may help you maintain that level of good health. However, if other conditions are affecting your health, you may choose less aggressive treatment so that you're less likely to experience many of the long-term detrimental effects of prostate cancer.

How much of a factor is your age?

Prostate cancer in your 80s is different from prostate cancer in your 40s. If you're in your later years, aggressive treatment may not extend your life and may not be warranted. You may prefer treatment that's less invasive and has less risk of severe complications.

A younger man may be willing to accept more aggressive treatment with more discomfort and significant side effects if that treatment offers a better chance of living longer. It's important to consider your general outlook on life. Do you think of yourself as young and active? If so, you may find it worthwhile to consider the more aggressive treatments, regardless of your chronological age.

How much will your chosen treatment affect your lifestyle?

Does the prospect of potential side effects — particularly impotence and urinary incontinence — bother you enough to sway your decision? Can your lifestyle accommodate, for example, a course of daily external beam radiotherapy?

Are you willing to commit to follow-up care?

Your condition needs to be monitored after treatment — and the less invasive your treatment is, probably the more important that monitoring becomes. Are you willing to undergo routine blood tests, digital rectal exams, imaging and perhaps biopsies? Are you willing to schedule follow-up appointments with your doctor as necessary?

When treatment ends, will you continue to worry about recurrent cancer?

If you choose active surveillance, how will you feel knowing that untreated cancer cells remain in your body? If you choose radiation — either seed implants or external beam radiotherapy — will you

feel more confident that the cancer is under control or do you need the certainty of surgery?

How will your decision affect your relationship with your life partner?

If you're married or in a relationship, you may want to think about how your decision will affect your partner. It's your life, but both of you will have to live with your decision.

Treatment for cancer can be a life-changing event. An open, honest discussion before making a treatment decision can help you both cope with changes in your relationship if urinary or sexual dysfunction results.

Discuss the trade-offs between the short-term and long-term effects. Your partner can help you talk through the value you place on benefits and risks. Your decision has biological, psychological and social aspects, and may very well affect your sexual relationship and your daily life years after therapy is complete.

Is your doctor's experience and training unduly influencing your decision?

Make sure you and your doctor decide on the treatment that's right for you, not just the treatment that your doctor is trained in or has the most experience with.

How do you find a doctor who's skilled in a particular procedure?

Before deciding on a particular course of treatment, talk with a doctor who can help explain the complexity of the choices you're facing and one who will listen to your values and concerns about health-related quality-of-life issues. You may feel more comfortable making a decision after you've heard a second opinion.

Doctors who treat prostate cancer are urologists, radiation oncologists and medical oncologists. You may want to talk with a specialist in each of these areas because each may have a different opinion on how best to proceed. If you choose a treatment option other than active surveillance, select a doctor who has extensive experience with it.

In many cases, your primary care physician may be able to refer you to a specialist, or help you evaluate your options.

MAKING YOUR DECISION

You'll likely face uncertainties in deciding on the best treatment for you. The tools for measuring how aggressive your cancer is aren't perfectly accurate. And it may be difficult for your doctor to pinpoint the spread of cancerous cells to other parts of your body.

How well you're able to accept risk is another area of uncertainty. You may feel comforted that the risk of urinary incontinence is only 5% for a particular treatment. But after the procedure, you'll be either zero or 100% continent, and that's an uncertainty that no one can predict.

(For more on incontinence and other side effects, see Chapter 9.)

The best decisions come from taking time to gather all the information, thinking things over carefully, consulting with experts and participating in the decision-making process. Your family and friends, as well as your primary doctor, the rest of the medical team and other cancer survivors, can offer advice, support and encouragement. You don't have to make the decision alone.

The process may seem difficult, but you'll have made your decision based on a careful, honest appraisal of the facts. Whatever you decide, don't be discouraged. Prostate cancer is curable and even the most advanced cancer can be controlled, sometimes for many years.

ANSWERS TO YOUR QUESTIONS

I'm considering active surveillance. What's a typical schedule for active surveillance?

Active surveillance for prostate cancer is most often considered for men with low-risk prostate cancer, specifically those with a Gleason 6 score. It's been shown to be a reasonably safe method of monitoring prostate cancer given that these tumors tend to grow very slowly and have a very low probability of spreading outside the prostate.

Active surveillance doesn't mean watchful waiting, but instead involves continued monitoring of the disease with repeat

PSA testing and repeat biopsies at scheduled intervals. MRI can also be integrated into active surveillance protocols to more accurately evaluate suspicious lesions that could be clinically significant prostate cancer (a Gleason score of 7 or higher). If an MRI wasn't obtained before the initial biopsy, getting one before starting on active surveillance can help confirm that there's no concerning lesions that could be clinically significant prostate cancer.

Typically, active surveillance would involve a confirmatory biopsy one year from the time of your initial diagnosis to assess whether there's any increase in the grade of the cancer — specifically, the development of Gleason 7 or higher prostate cancer. A confirmatory biopsy is also important to make sure that an accurate diagnosis has been obtained, since the initial biopsy may have missed potential areas of higher-grade disease.

PSA testing may be done at 6-month intervals from the time of initial diagnosis. If there's a change in your PSA, another biopsy may be recommended earlier.

Following a confirmatory biopsy, the schedule for future biopsies varies based on several factors including your biopsy results, MRI findings, PSA trends, your age and your overall health. Generally, if no changes are found after the second biopsy, biopsies can then be performed on an extended schedule, such as every 2 years. However, it's important to discuss with your doctor what schedule is most appropriate for you.

Is surgery more difficult in some men?

Radical prostatectomy can be more challenging in men who are obese or who have an especially deep or narrow pelvis. A very large prostate also can be more challenging to remove. However, a skilled surgeon should be able to overcome these obstacles. In some cases, if there's a history of extensive abdominal surgery, open prostatectomy may be recommended over robotic surgery due to concerns about scar formation.

Isn't radiation harmful?

Radiation can be harmful to normal tissue if given in excess. That's why the amount you receive during any type of radiation therapy is precisely calculated and controlled to minimize damage to healthy cells.

Can the radioactive seeds work their way out of the prostate gland?

Occasionally some seeds can get into the urethra and be excreted in your urine. This generally doesn't cause problems. Seeds may also infrequently become dislodged and travel through the bloodstream to other parts of the body, typically the chest and lungs. The number of seeds that may migrate from the prostate is very small — less than 1% — and few side effects have been reported. A type of seed that's built into an absorbable strand is designed to reduce the chance that seeds will migrate.

Should I get a second opinion before making a decision?

If you feel confident in your doctor and are comfortable with your treatment plan, a second opinion may not be necessary. However, if you have concerns about your diagnosis, you don't feel confident in your doctor, or you don't feel comfortable with the proposed treatment, then you may want another opinion.

If you're considering all treatment options, reviewing these options with different specialists is recommended.

Advanced and recurrent cancer

8

How you and your doctor decide to treat your prostate cancer — and the challenges you'll face — depends on a very basic fact: Cancer that's detected early and remains within the prostate gland is often less aggressive and is curable. Cancer that has spread to tissues outside the prostate gland is generally more advanced and more difficult to treat. In some cases, the cancer can't be cured.

Advanced prostate cancer comes in two forms:
- **Locally advanced cancer.** The cancer has invaded structures beyond the "shell" (capsule) of the prostate gland, such as the seminal vesicles or surrounding tissues, but it hasn't spread to lymph nodes or bone (see pages 40-41).
- **Metastatic (stage IV) cancer.** The cancer has spread beyond the prostate gland to more distant areas, such as lymph nodes and bone (see pages 45-46).

Advanced cancer may not produce noticeable signs and symptoms, but those that appear most often include bone pain and weight loss.

In certain situations — when the cancer is locally advanced or confined to a few adjacent lymph nodes and a cure is still possible — surgery or radiation may be used to treat the cancer. Otherwise, advanced cancer is often treated with medication.

When prostate cancer becomes advanced, the focus of treatment may shift from curing the cancer to therapies that can help slow its growth and perhaps even shrink cancerous tumors. The goal is to try to mold the cancer so that it can be treated more like a chronic disease. Attention is also directed at relieving symptoms, including managing pain.

The fact that metastatic prostate cancer is more serious and potentially life-threatening isn't a reason to give up hope. There have been tremendous strides in the management of advanced cancer, and there are many treatment options that can allow you to live longer — often many years — and enjoy a high quality of life.

HORMONE THERAPY

The cornerstone of treatment for advanced prostate cancer is medications that shut off the production and activity of male sex hormones (androgens). Testosterone is the main male sex hormone responsible for masculine features and the development of male reproductive organs. Testosterone also supports the spread of prostate cancer. Prostate cancer cells are highly dependent on androgens for survival and growth.

Circulation of androgens throughout the body and around cancer cells in the prostate gland encourages the cancer cells to multiply. A way to slow the growth of the cancer is to drastically reduce or cut off the supply of androgens to cancer cells. This weakens the cells and ultimately leads to their death. Depriving prostate cancer of androgens is known as hormone therapy, or androgen-deprivation therapy (ADT).

To decrease androgen levels, two methods may be used: medications or surgical removal of the testicles. The goal of each approach is to:
- Stop the body's production of male sex hormones (androgens).
- Block androgens in circulation from getting into cancer cells.

Sometimes, a combination approach may be implemented to try to achieve both.

Hormone therapy is usually the first line of treatment for men with advanced prostate cancer. Among most men, medications are preferred to surgical removal of the testicles, what's called orchiectomy.

Hormone therapy is so effective at shrinking tumors that it also may be used in some early-stage prostate cancers, primarily in combination with other treatments such as cryotherapy and radiation therapy. Hormone therapy can reduce the size of large tumors, making it easier for other treatments to destroy them. After more aggressive treatment, hormone therapy also may help kill stray cells left behind at the tumor site. And it may benefit some men in which cancer is found in nearby lymph nodes during prostatectomy surgery.

It's important to remember, though, that hormone therapy by itself generally isn't curative. It must be used in combination with another form of treatment to effectively rid the prostate of cancer. In addition, over time the cancer may become resistant to hormone medications, making them ineffective.

Hormone therapy medications

The specific medication your doctor prescribes to treat your cancer will depend on several factors, including how aggressive the cancer is, its current location outside the prostate gland, how widespread it is, whether you're experiencing symptoms, side effects of the medication and your personal preferences.

GnRH agonists

These medications, called gonadotropin-releasing hormone agonists, act by shutting off the brain's production of a hormone called luteinizing hormone-releasing hormone (LHRH). This action halts the manufacture of male sex hormones within the testicles, thereby starving cancer cells.

More than 90% of male hormones, specifically testosterone, are produced by the testicles. GnRH agonists basically set up a chemical blockade, preventing the testicles from receiving messages from the brain to make testosterone. These messages are carried by special brain chemicals.

GnRH agonists are synthetic hormones similar to your brain's natural messengers. But instead of turning on the chemical switch to activate the message pathway, they turn it off. Your testicles never get the alert to produce testosterone.

GnRH agonists include:
- Goserelin (Zoladex).
- Histrelin (Supprelin LA).
- Leuprolide (Camcevi, Eligard, Fensolvi, Lupron).
- Triptorelin (Trelstar, Triptodur).

The medications are injected into muscle or under the skin. Their effects last for a month to a year, depending on which medication is used. You may receive an injection of a hormone medication for a few months, a few years or the rest of your life, depending on your situation. The most common dosing schedule calls for an injection once every 3 to 6 months.

GnRH antagonists

The medication degarelix (Firmagon) is known as a gonadotropin-releasing hormone (GnRH) antagonist. It also works in the brain, reducing testosterone levels by blocking signals from the brain to the testicles to produce testosterone. This medication acts more rapidly than GnRH agonists. Degarelix may be prescribed to keep the cancer from progressing until other treatments have time to work. Two injections are given initially, then monthly thereafter.

A newer GnRH antagonist called relugolix (Orgovyx) works in a similar fashion but is available in pill form, making it more convenient to use. Relugolix also has been shown to cause fewer effects on cardiovascular function.

Testicular surgery

Surgically removing the testicles (orchiectomy) to prevent the production of testosterone was once the standard treatment for advanced prostate cancer. Hormone-blocking drugs that produce a similar effect with use of chemicals have greatly reduced the use of this procedure. Today, orchiectomy is rarely performed.

You might consider testicular surgery if:
- You can't tolerate hormone drug therapy for health reasons unrelated to your prostate cancer.
- You aren't able to take daily medication as prescribed, or regularly visit the doctor's office for hormone injections.
- There's an urgent need to eliminate testosterone from the body — more quickly than medications can act.

Orchiectomy is generally performed as an outpatient procedure using local anesthesia. A small incision is made at the center of the scrotum, the pouch that holds the testicles. Each testicle is clipped from the spermatic cord and removed, with most of the cord left in place. Some men have an artificial implant placed into the scrotum during the operation to maintain a more natural appearance. In a variation of this procedure (subcapsular approach), tissue is removed from within each testicle, but the lining and cord structure are left behind, resulting in near-normal appearing testicles.

Benefits and risks

If your cancer has spread beyond the prostate gland, you may benefit from hormone therapy. You also may be a candidate for hormone therapy if you're receiving radiation therapy for cancer that hasn't spread (metastasized) beyond the prostate gland.

The advantages of hormone therapy are:
- It can slow the growth of the cancer and shrink tumors, reducing your symptoms and allowing you to live longer.
- When used in conjunction with other treatments, such as radiation therapy, it may weaken cancer cells, improving the effectiveness of other treatments.
- The medications may be stopped temporarily, allowing the return of normal hormone production.
- Newer medications can be taken orally.

Hormone therapy is associated with several side effects. They include:
- Fatigue.
- Weight gain, often as much as 10 to 15 pounds.
- Loss of bone and muscle mass, increasing risk of a bone fracture.
- Loss of sex drive.
- Impotence and erectile dysfunction.
- Hot flashes.
- Mood changes and depression.
- Breast enlargement, potentially requiring low-dose radiation to the chest.
- Liver damage, generally without symptoms.
- Increased risk of heart attack.
- With testicular surgery, a feeling of reduced masculinity.

Because hormone therapy may pose a higher risk of heart attack the first year or two after starting treatment, your doctor should carefully monitor your heart health and aggressively treat other conditions that may predispose you to a heart attack, such as high blood pressure, high cholesterol and smoking.

ADDITIONAL MEDICATIONS

Using hormone therapy to deprive prostate cancer cells of testosterone is generally effective for a few years, slowing or stopping tumor growth. Early on, cancer cells are sensitive to the depletion of testosterone, and PSA levels generally decrease. During this period, you may also notice an improvement in symptoms, such as reduced bone pain and improved urinary symptoms. This stage when hormone therapy is working effectively is referred to as metastatic castration-sensitive prostate cancer (mCSPC).

But the effects of hormone therapy often don't last. After a few years of ongoing treatment, the cancer becomes resistant to the medications, and it begins to thrive without male hormones. This is known as hormone-refractory prostate cancer (HRPC) or metastatic castration-resistant prostate cancer (mCRPC). Indications that the cancer is becoming resistant to hormone therapy often include a rising PSA level and re-emergence of symptoms such as bone pain.

Once resistance develops, additional medications are generally required to try to control the cancer.

Their aim is to reduce signaling within cancer cell pathways or cause prostate cancer cell death by dismantling the scaffolding of the cell.

Antiandrogens

Not all testosterone is produced in the testicles. Around 5% to 10% comes from the adrenal glands, which are located on top of each of your kidneys.

Medications known as antiandrogens suppress production of testosterone by the adrenal glands and they keep testosterone from acting on cancer cells by competing with and eventually crowding out testosterone for entrance into the cells.

Antiandrogens come in pill form. Depending on the drug you're prescribed, you'll need to take the medication up to three times a day. Older antiandrogens include the medications:
- Bicalutamide (Casodex).
- Flutamide.
- Nilutamide (Nilandron).

Newer antiandrogens more strongly block male hormones from binding with androgen receptors on cancer cells than do older forms of the drug. Newer antiandrogens include the medications:
- Abiraterone (Zytiga).
- Apalutamide (Erleada).
- Enzalutamide (Xtandi).
- Darolutamide (Nubeqa).

Use of antiandrogens in combination with hormone therapy often results in little or no testosterone getting to the cancer cells. This is known as a total androgen blockade. Combination therapy involving newer antiandrogens have been shown to improve survival rates among men with advanced prostate cancer.

Antiandrogens also may be used when first starting a GnRH agonist medication. Initially, GnRH agonists may boost androgen production for a short period before they shut it down. This temporary boost may cause the cancer to flare and worsen. Combining an antiandrogen with a GnRH drug prevents that flare.

Side effects

A unique side effect of antiandrogen medications is breast enlargement (gynecomastia), causing breast tenderness. If you're prescribed the medication abiraterone, you'll also need to take a steroid medication such as prednisone.

Abiraterone blocks the production of the steroid hormone cortisol from the adrenal glands and prednisone helps replace the lost cortisol.

Chemotherapy

The role and timing of chemotherapy in the treatment of advanced prostate cancer is evolving. For some cancers, chemotherapy may be part of first-line treatment. It's most often combined with hormone therapy to help slow the spread of the cancer.

Chemotherapy uses chemicals to destroy cancer cells. The chemotherapy agent used most often to treat advanced prostate cancer is docetaxel (Taxotere). It's given intravenously once every 3 weeks, along with steroid pills that are taken twice daily to boost the effectiveness of the chemotherapy and reduce the risk of an allergic reaction.

Another chemotherapy drug commonly used to treat prostate cancer is cabazitaxel (Jevtana), which is also taken with a steroid. The treatment is administered intravenously every 3 weeks.

Treatment with chemotherapy often will extend a person's survival by several months, depending on what point in the course of the disease it's given. In the past, chemotherapy was generally prescribed when the cancer was no longer responding to hormone therapy. Today, it's being used earlier in cancer treatment in combination with hormone therapy medications to improve survival. Chemotherapy also may relieve pain and other cancer symptoms.

Side effects

Unfortunately, chemotherapy has unpleasant side effects because anticancer drugs are toxic to healthy cells as well as to cancer cells. Common side effects may include hair loss, nausea, vomiting, fatigue, changes in bowel function and lowered resistance to infection.

The severity of side effects varies from person to person. Among some individuals, the side effects may be mild, while in others they're more pronounced.

CONTINUOUS VERSUS INTERMITTENT THERAPY

As mentioned earlier, depriving prostate cancer of male hormones (androgens) usually slows cancer growth and spread. But eventually, the cancer becomes resistant to androgen-deprivation therapy.

Researchers believe that continuous use of hormone medications may be the reason why the cancer adapts. Therefore, a common approach to hormone therapy has been to take breaks from the medication, with the hope of keeping the cancer from adjusting to testosterone loss, or at least slowing the process. This approach to treatment is known as intermittent androgen-deprivation therapy.

With intermittent therapy, you stop taking hormone medications when the prostate-specific antigen (PSA) level in your blood is low and remains steady. You resume the medications when your PSA rises again to a significant level. A potential benefit of intermittent androgen-deprivation therapy is that this approach allows side effects to ease. Among other things, with intermittent therapy you may more likely be able to resume sexual activity.

However, studies haven't demonstrated that intermittent therapy reduces the risk of developing castration-resistant cancer. Plus, the survival rate associated with intermittent therapy isn't superior to that of continuous therapy.

More recent studies suggest that earlier use of antiandrogen medications — rather than waiting for the cancer to become resistant — and earlier use of chemotherapy may be beneficial. All of this is impacting the management of advanced

IMMUNOTHERAPY TO FIGHT THE CANCER

Scientists and researchers are continually exploring new therapies that can improve survival rates among men with advanced prostate cancer. This includes immunotherapy drugs designed to help your immune system recognize and attack the cancer. Some immunotherapy medications being studied in the treatment of prostate cancer include the following.

Sipuleucel-T. With this treatment, immune cells are collected from your blood and taken to a laboratory where they're exposed to genetically engineered proteins that activate the immune cells to fight prostate cancer cells. The immune cells are then infused back into your body. This is done over three treatments spaced 2 weeks apart. Sipuleucel-T (Provenge) is most often prescribed for men whose cancer has become resistant to androgen-deprivation therapy. It may be used before or after chemotherapy.

Pembrolizumab. This medication was developed to treat cancers that harbor genetic mutations affecting programmed cell death. Pembrolizumab (Keytruda) is the first tissue-agnostic cancer therapy approved in the United States. Cancer cells can sometimes hide from your body's immune system. Pembrolizumab works by blocking a specific protein pathway, thereby preventing cancer cells from hiding and allowing your immune system to detect and fight the cancer.

PARP inhibitors. PARP stands for poly-ADP ribosome polymerase. It's a protein found in cells that helps damaged cells repair themselves, including cancer cells. PARP inhibitors destroy cancer cells by stopping the repair protein from doing its job. Two medications currently used in the treatment of prostate cancer are olaparib (Lynparza) and rucaparib (Rubraca). The medications are recommended for men with mutations (variants) in specific genes, including the BRCA1 and BRCA2 genes.

The ultimate goal is to develop an immunotherapy treatment that can one day prevent the development of prostate cancer. Cancer vaccines remain an active area of research.

cancer. Among men with significant cancer spread (high-volume metastasis) the chemotherapy drug docetaxel may be combined with hormone therapy early on in treatment. And men with low-volume metastatic disease may benefit from adding one of the newer antiandrogen medications to hormone therapy sooner rather than later.

The approach to treatment that you undergo — continuous or intermittent — is generally dependent on the specifics of your disease, the medications you're receiving, your doctor's preferences and yours. But make sure to discuss with your doctor the potential advantages of starting some medications earlier versus waiting for the cancer to become resistant.

RADIATION AND SURGERY

When prostate cancer is advanced, doctors generally don't use radiation therapy or surgery to treat the cancer. There are times, however, when a doctor may recommend radiation or surgery, especially if you have locally advanced cancer.

Metastatic cancer

When prostate cancer spreads beyond the prostate gland (metastatic cancer), radiation or surgery often aren't helpful. However, data suggests that in cases in which spread of the cancer is limited, administration of radiation to those sites may slightly improve survival. Data supporting surgery is less clear. If the

COMMON TREATMENTS FOR ADVANCED CANCER

- Abiraterone
- Apalutamide
- Ensalutamide
- Darolutamide
- Sipuleucel-T
- Cabazitaxel
- Radium 223

cancer is confined to a small number of lymph nodes within the pelvis, surgery to remove the lymph nodes may be considered in some cases. Surgery is usually followed by additional treatments, such as radiation therapy or cryotherapy. In specific situations, hormone therapy also may be recommended after surgery.

Locally advanced cancer

Cancer that's locally advanced has migrated beyond the shell (capsule) of the prostate gland but it hasn't spread (metastasized) to distant locations. Some men with locally advanced cancer may benefit from surgery to remove the prostate gland or radiation therapy to destroy cancer cells.

As opposed to metastatic cancer, surgery or radiation to treat locally advanced cancer still offers the possibility of a cure. However, additional therapies are often incorporated because the risk of recurrence is higher with locally advanced cancer compared with men whose cancer isn't advanced.

To achieve a cure or delay progression of the cancer to distant sites, treatment for locally advanced cancer generally includes a combination of therapies. Surgery may be followed by radiation therapy, hormone therapy or both. Use of radiation after surgery without evidence of disease is called adjuvant therapy. It's given to preempt possible cancer spread. Adjuvant radiation therapy after surgery has been shown to improve survival among men with locally advanced cancer and reduce the need for hormone therapy. Hormone therapy, however, may be necessary if cancer is discovered in the pelvic lymph nodes during prostate surgery. Studies have found its use may improve survival.

An alternative approach to adjuvant radiation therapy is to monitor your PSA level after surgery but not administer radiation unless your PSA begins to increase. This strategy, called salvage radiation, takes into account that many men with locally advanced disease are cured with surgery alone and administration of adjuvant radiation therapy after surgery subjects them to unnecessary radiation.

With salvage radiation, there isn't a specific PSA level at which radiation should be initiated if your PSA starts to increase, but research suggests beginning radiation earlier (at a lower PSA level) is better than later. Salvage radiation is often combined with a short course of hormone therapy.

After prostate surgery, your PSA level should decrease to less than .1 nanograms per milliliter (ng/mL) — referred to as an undetectable level. If just radiation is used, your PSA level should decrease, but it may not reach an undetectable level. It may range between 0 and 2 ng/mL and fluctuate over time, what's sometimes referred to as a "radiation bounce."

With either surgery or radiation, a rise in PSA may indicate a cancer recurrence. Treatment of recurrent cancer is discussed beginning on page 158.

RELIEVING CANCER PAIN

Prostate cancer in its early stages typically isn't painful. However, once the cancer has spread beyond the prostate gland to nearby bone — the pelvic bones and, eventually, the spine — it may produce intense pain. For reasons that aren't clear, prostate cancer cells often migrate to bone tissue as they spread.

You don't need to endure pain as you manage your cancer. There are effective methods for relieving prostate cancer pain. Many times, hormone therapy medications used to treat the cancer also help reduce pain associated with its spread. Your doctor may recommend other approaches.

Treating local pain

Sometimes prostate cancer pain is confined to a specific location in your body, such as your lower back. Options for treating confined (localized) pain include the following:

External beam radiotherapy

With this procedure, a high-energy radiation beam is focused on locations where the cancer has spread and is causing pain (for more on this therapy, see page 126). External beam radiotherapy requires careful, precise planning that targets the cancer and reduces damage to adjoining bone and tissue. Treatment is usually effective in completely or partially relieving symptoms.

Radioactive drugs

Doctors may consider radioactive drugs (radiopharmaceuticals) to help relieve symptoms when the cancer has spread to multiple sites in bone and it can't be treated with standard radiation therapy. The radioactive elements samarium (Quadramet), strontium (Metastron) and radium 223 (Xofigo) are used in this targeted approach.

A radioactive drug is injected into your bloodstream, which carries the radioactive element to your bones where it's absorbed. Cancerous bone tissue absorbs more of the radioactive substance than does healthy tissue — which helps concentrate most of the drug at the source of your pain. The radiation kills the cancer cells.

The effects of samarium and strontium can last for several weeks or months, and sometimes even a year. If you find these injections helpful, you may receive more than one, but usually no more frequently than once every two months.

Radium 223 (Xofigo) is the newest radiopharmaceutical for delivering targeted radiation. Radium 223 targets cancer that's spread to the bones with alpha particles (a type of radiation). The drug can be given before or after chemotherapy. In addition to relieving pain, studies show that among men whose cancer has spread to bone, treatment with radium 223 can extend survival compared with men treated only with pain medications. Radium 223 is given in six treatments, a month apart. It delivers very high amounts of therapy to the tumor and very little radiation to surrounding healthy bone.

Depending on the dose you receive and the element used, your urine may be radioactive the first few days after an injection of a radioactive drug and you must dispose of it in a hazardous waste container. Following treatment, your white blood cell and blood platelet counts may temporarily decrease, putting you at increased risk of an infection. Therefore, you'll likely undergo regular testing to monitor your blood counts.

Nerve block

With a nerve block, an anesthesiologist injects numbing analgesic drugs into nerves at the pain site. This procedure works especially well if your pain is in a specific area where nerves can be identified and targeted.

The key to pain relief is working with your doctor to find an effective treatment. This may involve trial-and-error testing. If your first choice doesn't work, try another option. Keep trying until you find a therapy that controls your pain adequately and allows you to rest and be comfortable.

Many people believe that pain is something they have to put up with — that it can't be controlled. That's not true. Effective treatments are available. It's just a matter of finding the right one.

Other people worry that they may appear weak if they can't handle pain on their own. This also is a misconception. Advanced prostate cancer can produce severe pain because of the way it spreads to bone, including the lower spine. Seeking relief from pain isn't a sign of weakness.

Cryoablation

This minimally invasive procedure can achieve good pain control by freezing cancerous tumors in bone or in surrounding tissue. (For more on this therapy, see page 135.)

Radiofrequency ablation

A procedure called radiofrequency ablation can provide safe, effective relief of severe cancer-related bone pain when other treatments have failed.

In this procedure, a thin needle is inserted through the skin and guided to a cancerous tumor using computerized tomography (CT) or ultrasound imaging. A high-frequency current that creates intense heat is delivered through wires (electrodes) to the tumor. The heat deadens cancerous tissue. The treatment may also destroy nerves in the region that carry pain messages from the tumor site.

Radiofrequency ablation isn't a permanent solution for pain relief. The nerves often grow back, and the procedure may need to be repeated.

Surgery

Sometimes surgery is required to fix a fracture that's developed where bone has become weakened due to cancer.

Treating general pain

Sometimes pain isn't limited to a specific location. It may occur across a broader region of your body. This is often referred to as general or systemic pain.

If you have pain related to cancer, try to rate your experience of it on a scale of 1 to 10 — with 1 being no pain and 10 being the worst pain imaginable (see the graph below). This will help you and your doctor assess the impact the pain is having on your life. Medications are often the first course of treatment for general pain.

Medications

If your pain is mild and no more bothersome than a headache, an over-the-counter pain reliever may be all you need to manage it. If your pain is more intense, your doctor may prescribe a stronger prescription medication.

Opioids (narcotics) are drugs that are commonly recommended to relieve cancer pain. Some opioids are natural compounds derived from the opium poppy plant, while others are synthetic.

Opioids include drugs such as codeine, fentanyl, hydromorphone, methadone, morphine and oxycodone.

Opioids produce many side effects including mild dizziness, drowsiness, sedation and unclear thinking. Other side effects may include fatigue, constipation, nausea and vomiting. Ask your doctor about ways to manage these effects while taking the drugs.

Opioids are powerful pain relievers. When taken in small amounts for short periods, they generally cause only minor side effects. But when opioids are taken in increasing doses for several weeks or months, the side effects can impair your ability to function in daily life. This can place your goal of adequate pain relief at odds with your goal of improved quality of life. You and your doctor need to work out the best approach when considering narcotic medications.

Another potent painkiller is tramadol. Like other opioids, this prescription

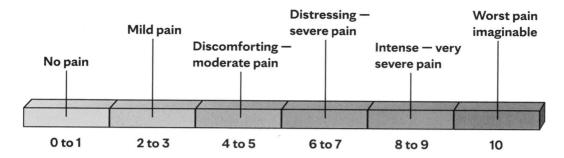

Pain scale Use this scale as a guide when describing your perceived level of pain to your doctor.

medication interferes with the transmission of pain signals. Tramadol also triggers the release of natural hormones in your body that help decrease your perception of pain. Side effects tend to be similar to those of other opioids.

IF YOUR CANCER RETURNS

Sometimes, prostate cancer can return. Most men who are treated for early-stage prostate cancer remain disease-free, but some experience a recurrence. When prostate cancer recurs, it means that not all the cancer was removed or destroyed — some cancer cells remained in the body after initial treatment. These cells have begun to grow to a degree where they can now be detected.

Recurrent cancer may develop for a variety of reasons. During surgery, small pockets of cancer cells may have escaped the prostate gland. Or a surgeon may not have been able to remove all the cancer within the prostate, leaving a few cells behind. With radiation therapy, efforts to avoid scatter radiation to nearby organs such as the bladder, urethra and rectum may have resulted in inadequate coverage of tissues surrounding the prostate, leaving some cancer cells behind.

Recurrence may happen weeks, months or years after an initial diagnosis. Sometimes, the cancer returns in the same location as the original tumor; other times, it recurs in a different location.

Identifying a recurrence

Most men who experience a cancer recurrence don't experience any symptoms, but their PSA level begins to rise. After surgery, a PSA level of less than 0.1 ng/mL signifies no cancer. When PSA levels begin to rise above this amount, it's an indication to doctors that the cancer may have come back, especially when the level reaches 0.2 ng/mL.

WHAT ABOUT COMPLEMENTARY AND ALTERNATIVE THERAPIES?

Some people look to less conventional methods for pain relief — what's commonly referred to as complementary and alternative medicine, or integrative medicine. These therapies range from massage and meditation to acupuncture and tai chi. Use of alternative therapies has become more popular as people seek greater control of their own health.

Under careful supervision, some alternative and complementary therapies may be beneficial in helping control your pain. See Chapter 12 for information on practices to manage pain.

There are situations, however, when a PSA level of 0.2 ng/mL or higher after radical prostatectomy surgery does not signify cancer. The increase may be due to noncancerous (benign) tissue in the prostate gland that wasn't removed during surgery. Because of this, an alternative threshold often used is 0.4 ng/mL or above. When PSA reaches this level, it's more likely to signify cancer than benign tissue.

After radiation therapy, PSA rarely drops to an undetectable level. There's usually some persistence in elevation, often in the range of 0 to 2 ng/mL. Following radiation, most men develop a specific range in which their PSA fluctuates. A PSA level that starts to exceed your normal range may represent a recurrence of the cancer.

Once PSA levels begin to rise, doctors are challenged by the fact that standard imaging tests generally aren't able to identify where the cancer has recurred. So, doctors often don't know if the cancer is located within the pelvic area or has established itself at more distant sites. Therefore, determining the best course of treatment can be difficult.

For cancer that has recurred within the pelvis, salvage radiation therapy may be the most appropriate treatment to eradicate the cancer. If the recurrence is outside the pelvis in more distant sites, medication — often hormone therapy

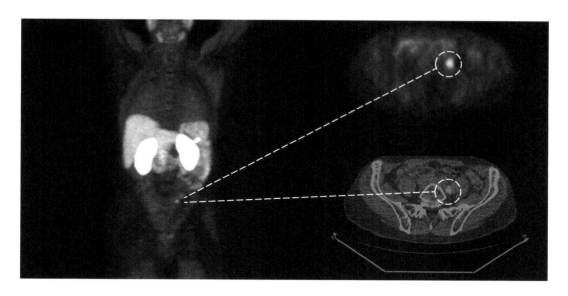

Choline C-11 PET For this imaging, a small amount of chemical tracer (radionuclide) is injected into a vein just before the scan is done. Prostate cancer cells in your body readily absorb this tracer, as shown by the colorful areas that are marked. This type of imaging is particularly helpful for detecting sites of cancer recurrence.

combined with an antiandrogen — is generally most effective.

To help doctors identify the location of recurrence, more sensitive imaging tests are emerging (see pages 106-108) that are better able to detect prostate cancer cells and identify small areas of recurrence that would not have been identified with conventional imaging.

Treating recurrent cancer

Treatment of recurrent cancer depends primarily on the location of the cancer. It's important to note that when cancer returns within the pelvis and it hasn't spread to other areas, a cure may still be possible. That's why knowing where the cancer is located is crucial.

Recurrent cancer after prostatectomy surgery that's confined to the pelvis is often treated with radiation — what's often called salvage radiation therapy — and possibly hormone therapy. External beam radiation is paired with advanced imaging to precisely deliver multiple beams of high-dose radiation to targeted tissues at risk for cancer recurrence, including the space the prostate gland occupied before it was removed. Hormone therapy may be used in conjunction with radiation to increase the chances of a cure.

If your cancer was initially treated with radiation and the recurrence appears to be confined to the prostate gland, you may be a candidate for a salvage procedure. In select cases, a surgeon may consider surgery to remove the prostate gland, the seminal vesicles and, often, surrounding lymph nodes. This is referred to as salvage prostatectomy.

Ablation therapy is another possible treatment for recurrent cancer after radiation. Ablation uses thermal energy — extreme heat or cold — to destroy targeted cancerous tissue.

In case of extreme heat, sound waves known as high-intensity focused ultrasound (HIFU) are used to destroy cancer cells. A procedure known as cryoablation uses extreme cold to freeze cancer cells. (For more on ablation therapy, see Chapter 7.) Another potential salvage treatment is brachytherapy, in which rice-size radioactive seeds (pellets) are injected into the prostate gland in an attempt to kill cancer cells (see page 130).

For cancer located outside the pelvic area, a variety of treatments may be considered, including hormone therapy, chemotherapy and immunotherapy.

The type of therapy you may receive is dependent on a variety of factors — the characteristics of your cancer, your overall health, previous treatments and imaging results.

ANSWERS TO YOUR QUESTIONS

Can hormone therapy control prostate cancer for several years?

Yes. Many cancers adapt and learn to grow without the presence of hormones within 1 to 3 years. But for some men, hormone therapy can control the spread of cancer for up to 10 years.

Will hormone therapy affect my voice or outward appearance?

No. Both your voice and outward appearance should remain the same.

Do I need to worry about becoming addicted to painkillers?

Many pain medications can be used effectively over many months and years without the danger of addiction. In cases of advanced cancer, the relief of pain, not addiction, is often your primary concern.

I had surgery to treat my cancer and now my PSA level is detectable and rising. Does this mean I have metastatic disease?

It's important to remember that prostate cancer recurrence comes in many forms. A rising PSA level alone isn't synonymous with metastatic disease. In fact, many times when imaging tests are performed in an individual with a rising PSA level, a site of disease recurrence can't be found. This means the recurrence may be within the pelvis near where the prostate gland was located before its removal.

The average time between early indications of a rising PSA level and the development of metastatic disease is approximately 5 to 8 years. A significant amount of time may elapse before imaging is able to identify an area of cancer spread within the body. It's important to understand that while a rising PSA level gener-

ally precedes the development of metastatic disease, it doesn't necessarily indicate the onset of sudden, severe disease. In fact, some individuals with other health problems may die of other causes before metastatic cancer develops.

What kind of tests are used to identify possible disease recurrence?

Traditionally, bone scans and computerized tomography (CT) scans were used when PSA levels began to increase. However, these tests aren't very sensitive in identifying early cancer recurrence, particularly among men with low PSA values. More recently, there's been an increase in use of positron emission tomography (PET) scans in the identification of recurrent cancer. Specific scans that may be used include PSMA PET, choline PET and fluciclovine PET.

9

Coping with complications

Prostate cancer is often a double blow. The first blow is that you have cancer. The second comes when you find out that treating the cancer may leave you with urinary changes, erectile dysfunction, or both. In fact, the possibility of such side effects can be more difficult for some men to accept than the cancer itself.

Side effects such as erectile dysfunction, incontinence and bowel disorders can erode feelings of self-worth. They can make you feel less in control and less masculine. They can affect your quality of life and your independence. Plus, acknowledging such problems, even in private discussions with members of your health care team, may feel awkward.

It's true that erectile dysfunction and urinary and bowel changes are common

side effects of prostate cancer, and that these conditions affect many men. But it's also important to understand that when these side effects occur as a part of prostate cancer treatment, they're often temporary. And even in situations when they are permanent, they don't need to be devastating.

To help manage these common complications, it's important to be open and honest with your doctor and health care team about the issues you're experiencing. These individuals can provide support and advice on possible solutions.

Various treatments are available that can help you effectively manage the complications of cancer treatment. This in turn can help you once again enjoy a good quality of life.

MANAGING INCONTINENCE

Urinary incontinence is the inability to control the flow of urine from your bladder, resulting in accidental and untimely leakage. Incontinence may be associated with an underlying condition, or it may be the byproduct of treatment — procedures or medications — used to treat a particular condition.

With prostate cancer, use of surgery, radiation therapy, or ablation to remove or destroy the cancer commonly leads to incontinence.

Most often, the incontinence is only temporary. Long-term incontinence after prostate cancer treatment is uncommon. But when it persists, it can be extremely frustrating and embarrassing. You may stop exercising, stop going out socially or even resist the urge to laugh because you're afraid of accidentally wetting yourself.

Like many men, you may be too embarrassed to ask for help. Perhaps you think that having incontinence is simply the price to pay for having prostate cancer — and that you'll just have to learn to live

Bladder relaxed   **Bladder contracted**

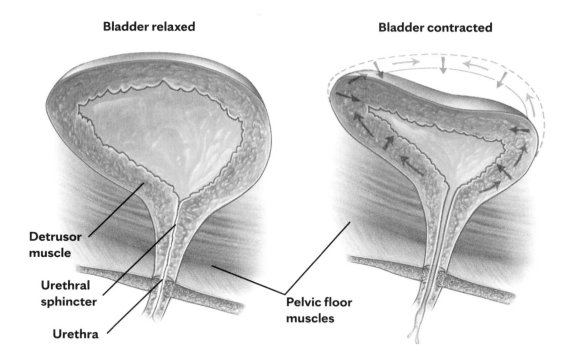

Detrusor muscle

Urethral sphincter

Urethra

Pelvic floor muscles

The detrusor muscle surrounds the bladder. When it contracts (right), and when the urethral sphincter at the base of the bladder relaxes, urine flows through the urethra.

with it. That's not true. Incontinence often can be successfully treated.

For your urinary system to function properly, a complex network of muscles and nerves must work together harmoniously. Except when you're urinating, your bladder muscle stays relaxed so that it can expand to store urine. The relaxed bladder is supported by muscles located in your lower pelvis (pelvic floor muscles). Your bladder and pelvic floor muscles communicate to help hold urine in the bladder without leaking.

Also helping control urine flow is a ring of muscle at the base of the bladder called the internal sphincter. The sphincter's ability to contract around the urethra to close it, or relax to open it, also depends on involuntary pelvic floor muscles.

Treatments for prostate cancer can affect the pelvic floor muscles and the nerves that control them, producing incontinence. Often, though not always, the incontinence is temporary, and healing occurs over weeks or months as the muscles slowly regain their strength and their ability to control urine flow.

Types of incontinence

Urinary incontinence is divided into four major categories:

Stress

This type of incontinence is caused by physical stress on the bladder. Urine leaks occur with bursts of activity that put intense pressure on the bladder, such as exercising, lifting a heavy object, swinging a golf club, sneezing or laughing. This form of incontinence is most common after surgery to remove the prostate gland.

Urge

With this type, you feel an immediate, intense urge to urinate with little warning, and you may wet yourself before getting to the bathroom. This happens due to an overactive bladder, which contracts too often and at inappropriate times trying to expel the urine. Your brain gets the message that you have to go — now! The need to urinate frequently, including several times throughout the night, also is common with this type. Urge incontinence may develop after radiation therapy due to irritation associated with the scatter of radiation to the bladder.

Overflow

Overflow incontinence occurs when you're unable to empty your bladder completely, leading to urine backup. The backup creates pressure that exceeds your bladder's capacity to hold fluid. You frequently dribble small amounts of urine throughout the day. You may feel as if you never completely empty your bladder, or that you need to empty your bladder but can't. When you try to urinate, you may have trouble getting started and may produce only a weak urine stream.

This type is common in men with bladder damage, an obstructed urethra, urethral narrowing (stricture) and some prostate problems. It also may develop when metastatic cancer injures spinal cord nerves that help squeeze the bladder.

Mixed

This is a combination of two or more types of incontinence, typically stress incontinence and urge incontinence. You experience signs and symptoms of both, but usually one type is more bothersome than the other. The causes of the two types may or may not be related. If you've had surgery for an enlarged prostate gland, you can develop mixed incontinence.

Treatment

For most men, stress incontinence after prostate surgery is temporary and symptoms diminish as normal bladder control gradually returns over a period of weeks to months. After prostate surgery you'll likely need to wear a catheter for 1 to 2 weeks while swollen tissues heal. Incontinence may occur when the catheter is removed and while the pelvic floor muscles are still weak.

While you regain control of urine flow, you may need to wear absorbent pads or protective underwear. Most men see a noticeable reduction in urine leakage within a short time, as the pelvic floor muscles and nerves strengthen.

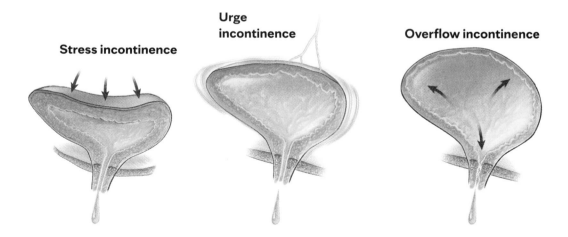

Stress incontinence   **Urge incontinence**   **Overflow incontinence**

With stress incontinence (left), urine leaks when you exert pressure on the bladder when coughing, sneezing, laughing or lifting. With urge incontinence (center), the bladder muscle contracts too often, signaling your brain that you have to urinate. It's characterized by a sudden, involuntary loss of bladder control. Overflow incontinence (right) is characterized by frequent urination or dribbling of urine.

For a minority of men, incontinence becomes chronic. In these situations, other treatments may be needed to manage the problem, including behavior therapies, medications, urinary devices and surgery. Your doctor will likely suggest the least invasive treatment first and move to other options if needed.

Behavior therapies

A common therapy used in the treatment of incontinence is bladder training.

Bladder training involves teaching your bladder new habits of urinating on a set schedule instead of waiting for the urge to go. You urinate on a planned basis — usually every hour or so at the start, and then building to longer intervals — to retrain the bladder. This makes it possible for you to gain control over frequent urges and allows your bladder enough time to fill properly.

Behavior therapies also include adjusting your dietary habits, for example, learning to avoid alcohol, caffeine and certain

WHAT'S A URETHRAL STRICTURE?

A urethral stricture is a narrowing of the urethra. It may occur in men who've undergone surgery or other procedures to treat benign prostatic hyperplasia (BPH), as well as radical prostatectomy or radiation therapy to treat prostate cancer.

When your prostate is removed, the upper portion of the urethra is reattached to the bottom of your bladder. This restores the urinary channel, which previously had been surrounded by the prostate. Sometimes, scar tissue forms in the area where the urethra and bladder were reattached, causing the urethra to narrow. This is more common when radiation is required after surgery.

Among men who receive radiation therapy to treat prostate cancer, the radiation may damage healthy urethral tissue, resulting in scarring and narrowing, also known as a stricture.

Usually, the first line of treatment is to stretch the urethra by dilating it with a thin instrument that's inserted into the urethra. This is the simplest and safest approach. Occasionally, a stricture needs to be opened surgically. In some people, these procedures must be repeated more than once because of renarrowing. If the stricture is severe, your doctor may suggest laser treatment to vaporize the scar tissue.

acidic foods that irritate your bladder. For some men, drinking fewer liquids before bedtime can reduce or eliminate nightly trips to the bathroom. Losing weight also may improve the problem.

Some simple tips also can be helpful. For example, with stress incontinence, crossing your legs when you feel something like a sneeze coming on may prevent urine from leaking.

Pelvic floor muscle training

This form of treatment involves doing exercises commonly referred to as Kegel exercises to strengthen weak urethral sphincter and pelvic floor muscles — the muscles that help control urination and defecation. Your doctor may recommend that you do these exercises regularly to treat incontinence. (For more on these exercises, see page 168.)

With Kegels, it can be difficult to know at first whether you're contracting the right muscles and in the right manner. In general, you should sense a feeling of your penis pulling in slightly toward your body when you squeeze.

You can use Kegel exercises when you experience a strong urge to urinate or when you're trying to wait longer to go to the bathroom. While you're contracting the muscles, try to think of something other than going to the bathroom. When you feel the urge lessen somewhat, walk normally to the bathroom.

Kegel exercises are the most effective treatment for mild to moderate incontinence. After several months of doing

TESTS FOR INCONTINENCE

If you have urinary incontinence, your doctor may perform a series of diagnostic tests to determine the type of incontinence you have and how best to treat it. These tests may include:

- **Video urodynamic tests.** Use of X-rays or ultrasound to capture images of the bladder while it fills and empties.
- **Cystoscopy.** Examination of the inner surface of your urinary tract and your urinary sphincter muscle by inserting a thin, flexible tube equipped with a light and lens into your urethra.
- **Cystometry.** Measurement of varying pressure levels as your bladder fills with, and then releases, urine.
- **Uroflowmetry.** Measurement of the force of your urine flow, including the amount you release, how fast it leaves your penis, and how long it takes to empty your bladder.

these exercises correctly, muscle strength should gradually improve, and you'll gain greater urinary control.

Medications

Sometimes, urinary incontinence can be corrected with the help of medication. Medications are often used in combination with behavior techniques. Medications are generally most effective for men with urge incontinence from an overactive bladder. There currently aren't any medications to treat stress incontinence.

Drugs that may be prescribed to treat incontinence include anticholinergic (antispasmodic) drugs that help relax muscles and calm an overactive bladder. This class of drugs includes darifenacin, oxybutynin (Ditropan XL), solifenacin

---

HOW TO DO KEGEL EXERCISES

To perform these exercises, first you need to locate your pelvic floor muscles. Imagine that you're trying to avoid passing gas in public. The muscles that you use to keep the gas from escaping are your pelvic floor muscles.

Once you've identified your pelvic floor muscles, get into a comfortable sitting or standing position. Then firmly tense the muscles. Try to pull in your penis and squeeze your anus without tightening your buttocks or your belly. Hold the contraction for a count of five (5 seconds) and then relax the muscles. If you're not able to hold the contraction for 5 seconds, try to hold it for a count of three (3 seconds), and gradually increase the time up to 10 seconds. Rest for 10 seconds between each contraction.

Aim to perform 10 repetitions at least three times a day, and practice the exercises in different positions, including while sitting and standing. Some men find it helpful to do the exercises while sitting on the toilet seat. It's recommended that you do them before bedtime with an empty bladder. This allows your muscles to rest afterward while you sleep.

Kegel exercises will get easier the more often you do them. Eventually, you might include a set while you perform routine tasks, for example, as you commute to work. You can also vary your technique. You might try sets of mini-Kegels — count quickly to 10 or 20, contracting and relaxing the pelvic floor muscles every time you say a number. Your health care team may have additional suggestions.

(Vesicare), tolterodine (Detrol) and trospium.

Side effects of anticholinergic drugs may include dry mouth, blurred vision and constipation. To combat dry mouth, you may be tempted to drink more water, but this may further affect your incontinence. Instead, your doctor may recommend sucking on a piece of candy or chewing gum to produce more saliva. The medications oxybutynin and tolterodine are available in extended-release forms, and oxybutynin comes as a skin patch (Gelnique, Oxytrol). They may have fewer side effects than the standard forms.

Other medications used to treat incontinence include mirabegron (Myrbetriq) and vibegron (Gemtesa), which belong to a class of drugs known as beta-3 adrenergic agonists. The medications improve the storage capacity of the bladder by relaxing the bladder muscle during filling. Imipramine (Tofranil) is an older antidepressant that may occasionally be prescribed to help treat bladder dysfunction related to spinal cord injury.

For men experiencing urge incontinence, botulinum toxin type A (Botox) may be injected into the muscles of the bladder to treat incontinence associated with nerve damage. Botox causes the bladder to relax, increasing its storage capacity and reducing incontinent episodes. Treatment may need to be repeated. Occasional urinary retention and infection can result.

If your incontinence is due to a urinary tract infection or an inflamed prostate, your doctor can successfully treat the problem with antibiotics.

Surgical approaches

If less invasive therapies aren't working and you continue to experience leakage problems for at least a year without signs of improvement, your doctor may suggest a more invasive procedure.
- **Sling procedure.** With this procedure, a section of synthetic meshlike tape is used to compress the urethra against the pubic bone. This is done through an incision in the area between the scrotum and rectum (perineum). A male sling is used to treat mild to moderate stress incontinence. Because the procedure is minimally invasive, recovery time is generally short.
- **Surgery.** Sometimes it's necessary to surgically remove blockages in the urinary tract, improve the position of the bladder neck or add support to the bladder or weakened pelvic floor muscles.
- **Artificial sphincter.** An artificial sphincter is a small device that's particularly helpful for men with urethral sphincters weakened from treatment of prostate cancer or an enlarged prostate gland. A small, doughnut-shaped device is implanted around the neck of the bladder (see the illustration on page 170). Its fluid-filled ring keeps your urethral sphincter closed until you're ready to urinate. To urinate, you press a valve implanted in your scrotum that causes the ring to deflate and allows urine from your bladder to be released. Once your

bladder is empty, the device reinflates over the next few minutes. The device isn't activated until the area where it was placed has time to heal. This treatment can cure or greatly improve incontinence in most men.

- **Sacral nerve stimulation.** With this procedure, a device (stimulator) that resembles a pacemaker is implanted under the skin in your abdomen. A wire from the device is connected to the sacral nerve at the base of the spinal cord that connects to the bladder. The stimulator emits electrical impulses that interfere with the abnormal messaging between the brain and sacral nerve that is causing an overactive bladder.
- **Bulking agents.** Sometimes urinary incontinence may be treated by injecting substances into tissues and muscles to help support the bladder and other urinary organs. This approach is generally prescribed if medications haven't been successful and surgery isn't an option or you'd like to avoid surgery. Unfortunately, bulking agents to treat stress incontinence are rarely effective or provide only modest benefits. An injection of a bulking material tightens the seal of the urinary sphincter by bulking up the surrounding tissue. However, many bulking agents lose their effectiveness over time and repeat injections are often needed.

Absorbent pads and catheters

While waiting for other measures to work or in situations when treatment is ineffective, you may need to rely on absorbent pads to manage your incontinence. Most absorbent products are no more bulky than normal underwear, and they can be worn easily under everyday clothing. They can be purchased in drugstores, supermarkets and medical supply stores.

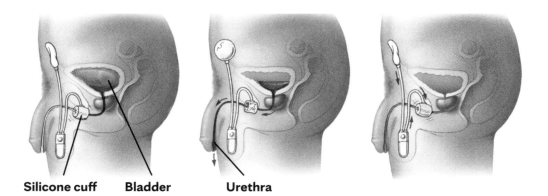

Silicone cuff   **Bladder**   **Urethra**

Artificial sphincter An artificial sphincter uses a tiny silicone cuff placed around the urethra to treat incontinence. When inflated, the cuff squeezes the urethra, preventing urine from leaking. To urinate, you deflate the cuff, allowing urine to pass.

A catheter is a thin tube that's inserted in the urethra. It allows urine to drain from the bladder. A couple of different approaches may be used.

- A medical provider may teach you how to drain your bladder using self-catheterization, in which you insert a thin, flexible tube through your urethra and into your bladder.
- A type of catheter called an indwelling catheter, which remains in place continuously, may be used. A bag attached to the catheter collects urine.
- A condom catheter is a special condom that fits over the penis and is attached to a tube that collects urine. It doesn't require an internal catheter to be placed in the urethra.

Side effects of catheter use can include urinary tract infections and skin irritation. Proper sterilizing techniques can prevent these problems from occurring.

MANAGING ERECTILE DYSFUNCTION

Temporary or permanent loss of erectile function after prostate cancer treatment is very common. Even in cases of excellent nerve preservation during surgery, it's unusual to return to your original level of erectile function. The need for additional treatment after surgery also may impact erectile function.

Erectile dysfunction that results from prostate cancer treatment may be related to several different factors. Prostate cancer itself may cause changes to the blood vessels and nerves responsible for normal erectile function. Surgery or whole prostate cryotherapy often result in temporary or permanent injury to the nerves that help produce erections. Radiation therapy may damage the nerves, blood vessels or tissue in the penis. Hormone therapy can have widespread effects on sexual health, including reduced erectile function, difficulty achieving an orgasm and decreased sexual desire (libido).

Although you may view erectile dysfunction as an embarrassing problem, it's important that you talk to your doctor. In most cases, erectile dysfunction can be successfully treated. Studies have found, however, that it's best to address the problem early. The sooner you seek help for erectile dysfunction the better your chances of improving your sexual health, including achieving erections.

Your doctor will take into consideration the cause and severity of your dysfunction in determining the best course of treatment. Your treatment plan may include a combination of approaches.

Oral medication

Prescription medications, in tablet or capsule form, are typically the first line of treatment for erectile dysfunction. They include the drugs:

- Avanafil (Stendra).
- Sildenafil (Viagra).
- Tadalafil (Cialis).
- Vardenafil (Levitra, Staxyn).

All four medications work in much the same way. These drugs, chemically known as phosphodiesterase-5 inhibitors, enhance the effects of nitric oxide, a naturally occurring chemical that relaxes muscles in the penis. This increases the amount of blood flow and allows a natural erection sequence to take place.

The medications don't automatically produce an erection. You'll still require sexual stimulation — physical and emotional — for the erection to occur. Regardless of the situation, many men experience improvement in erectile function after this treatment.

Though they're similar in many ways, the medications have differences as well. They vary in dosage, how long they work and side effects. The medications might not treat your erectile dysfunction immediately. You might need to work with your doctor to find the right medication and dosage.

Consult your doctor to determine the best approach for you. Individual dosages may need adjusting. You may need to alter your schedule to take the medication. Your doctor will probably start you on an average dose and increase or decrease the amount you take, depending on your individual response to the medication.

Not all men can or should take these medications to treat erectile dysfunction. Tell your doctor if you:
• Take nitrate drugs for angina, such as nitroglycerin (Nitro-Dur, Nitrostat, others), isosorbide mononitrate (Monoket) and isosorbide dinitrate (BiDil, Isordil).

• Have heart disease or heart failure.
• Have very low blood pressure (hypotension).

Side effects of the medications include facial flushing, which generally lasts no more than 5 to 10 minutes. You might also experience nasal congestion, mild headache, stomach upset, visual changes and backache. These effects generally subside a few hours after taking the drug.

Intraurethral therapy

If oral medications fail to help, another option involves placing a suppository medication into the opening of the penis (urethra) using a special applicator. Intraurethral alprostadil (Muse) is a synthetic version of the natural hormone prostaglandin E. This treatment directly relaxes the muscles in the penis and results in an erection even in cases where the nerves responsible for erections were removed or damaged. After placement, it generally takes about 10 minutes for the medication to take effect.

Intraurethral therapy may result in some pain or a sensation of penile burning, minor bleeding, and the formation of fibrous tissue inside the penis.

Self-injection therapy

With this method you use a fine needle to inject medication into the penis. Because the needle used is very fine, pain at the injection site is usually minor. The medication most often used is alprostadil

(Caverject, edex). Sometimes medications used for other conditions, such as the drugs papaverine and phentolamine, may be used on their own or in combination with another drug. Self-injected medications produce an erection directly without need for stimulation.

This approach is often effective in cases where the nerves have been resected or damaged with prior prostate treatments. If started early enough, the medications may be effective for years and may result in an erection that more closely resembles the one that was present prior to prostate treatment.

The injection is performed near the base of the shaft of the penis and often achieves an erection within 10 to 15 minutes. No more than one injection should be used within a 24-hour period, and you should contact your doctor

before combining this medicine with other therapies for erectile dysfunction. Serious complications, including infection and a prolonged erection (priapism), are rare.

Penis pumps

These devices use vacuum pressure to draw blood into your penis. You place an airtight, plastic tube over your penis that's attached to a hand-powered or battery-powered pump. The pump draws air out of the plastic tube. This creates a vacuum effect, which pulls blood into your penis. The increased blood flow produces an erection.

When you achieve an adequate erection, you slip an elastic ring around the base of

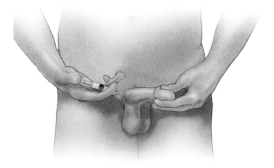

Self-injection therapy This method introduces the drug alprostadil directly to the penis to increase blood flow and cause an erection. It takes several minutes to take effect.

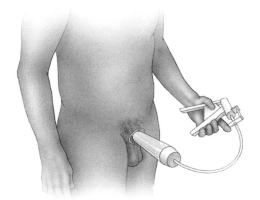

Penis pump These devices use a pump and vacuum pressure to draw blood into the penis and create an erection. An elastic ring placed at the base of the penis keeps it erect.

your penis to hold in the blood and keep the penis firm. The ring should be removed within 30 minutes to restore normal blood flow. You could possibly damage penile tissue if you keep the penis erect for a longer period.

Temporary side effects include a bluish appearance of the penis, reduced penile sensation, restricted ejaculation and a cold penis. Bruising of the penis also is a possible side effect. For men who've had prostate surgery, the pump may cause

INTIMACY WITHOUT INTERCOURSE

For most couples, sexuality and intimacy are delicately balanced. Intercourse can lead to physical, emotional and, at times, a deeply spiritual experience. It can be a way to connect with one another during times of joy and sadness. But there are many other pathways to achieve a similar level of intimacy.

Sexual intercourse may well have been something that was of value to you and was tied to your personal identity. If the ability to have intercourse is lost or diminished, you may feel alone, unwanted, unattractive and powerless. You may worry about maintaining your relationship or that your partner might seek sex outside the relationship. This may be especially true if you aren't able to talk about the situation and work through it.

To maintain intimacy in your relationship, try to open your heart to your partner and find different ways to be intimate — sexually, sensually or spiritually. If you're willing to invest in this growth together, you may find an even deeper connection than you had before. This may involve re-experiencing some of the same phases you enjoyed early in your relationship that you've since skipped over to get to intercourse.

Everything from kissing, cuddling and massage, to the types of things you used to do as foreplay, can be satisfying within the context of a loving relationship. Touch is often very personal, but each person's needs may be different and change over time. Lie next to your partner and be open in every way.

Use warmth and companionship as your guide to finding the next steps. Talk about what each of you wants and needs for closeness. Be considerate. Try to build each other up. Laugh together and work at being more in rhythm as a couple. Most important, understand that it's still possible to have a dynamic, growing and totally fulfilling relationship without intercourse.

urine to be pulled out of the penis and into the device.

Penile implants

This treatment involves surgically placing devices into both sides of the penis. These implants consist of either inflatable or malleable (bendable) rods. Inflatable devices allow you to control when and how long you have an erection. The malleable rods keep your penis firm but bendable.

Penile implants are usually not recommended until other methods have been tried. Implants have a high degree of satisfaction among men who have tried more conservative therapies that were unsuccessful. As with any surgery, there's a risk of complications, such as infection.

OTHER SEXUAL CONCERNS

Treatment for prostate cancer can result in a number of sexual dysfunctions. Along with erectile dysfunction, other conditions that may develop include orgasmic dysfunction, leakage of urine with orgasm, loss of penile length or penile curvature (Peyronie's disease). The extent of these dysfunctions depends on the treatment that you receive or specific factors relating to the procedure.

Orgasmic and ejaculatory dysfunction

Many men experience orgasm and ejaculation changes after prostate cancer treatment. In particular, you may notice significantly reduced or absent ejaculation after orgasm. Reduced ejaculation after surgery is often a result of removal (resection) of the tubes that drain ejaculatory fluid into the urethra. Absent ejaculation after radiation and ablation may be associated with scarring of the ejaculatory ducts. Another cause may be decreased pleasure from orgasm, which may be related to low testosterone levels.

Another common occurrence after prostatectomy is urine leakage with orgasm. This condition, called climacturia, often improves spontaneously over time. To reduce the amount of leakage, it's recommended that you empty your bladder before engaging in intercourse. If the symptoms remain, a penile clamp or constriction band may be applied. Medications are often of limited benefit and cause side effects.

Reduced penile length

Some men who undergo prostate cancer treatment may complain of reduced penile length. Some prostate treatments can lead to a reduction of 1 to 2 centimeters in penile length. Additional loss may occur over time among men who are unable to achieve an erection.

You may also notice an increase in the fat pad located above the penis. This may give the appearance of a shortened penis and reduce its functional length.

Penile traction therapy may be used to preserve or increase the length of the penis. This involves stretching the penis for a period of time with a self-applied mechanical device to improve penile length, curvature and deformity.

Depending on the device, traction therapy may need to be applied for as little as 30 minutes to as much as 3 to 8 hours a day to achieve benefits. The effectiveness of treatment may also depend on the specific device used. Although vacuum erection devices also help improve penile length, penile traction may be preferred in certain cases, partic-

WHAT ABOUT TESTOSTERONE THERAPY?

After treatment of prostate disease, some men are worried about low testosterone levels. Testosterone deficiency syndrome — also known as androgen deficiency or low T — may be marked by erectile dysfunction, decreased beard and body hair growth, decreased muscle mass, fatigue and decreased sex drive.

To combat the problem, men are typically treated with testosterone. But is testosterone therapy safe if you have a prostate condition, especially prostate cancer?

Studies evaluating the impact of testosterone replacement on various prostate-related outcomes have been inconsistent and contradictory. Some studies suggest an increased risk of having an elevated prostate-specific antigen (PSA) — requiring a prostate biopsy — or of experiencing urinary symptoms. Other studies have concluded the opposite.

Research has consistently demonstrated that testosterone replacement doesn't increase the risk of developing prostate cancer. However, there's debate on the potential risks and benefits of testosterone therapy in men with existing early-stage prostate cancer or men with treated prostate cancer. And caution is still advised for men with more advanced prostate cancer because of the potential risk of increasing cancer spread.

If you're considering testosterone therapy, talk to your doctor about its risks and benefits. Keep in mind that in addition to stimulating the growth of existing prostate cancer, testosterone therapy may also contribute to noncancerous growth of the prostate, sleep apnea, enlarged breasts, reduced sperm production, blood clot formation and increased risk of a heart attack.

ularly in men with urinary incontinence, who are less able to use vacuum devices.

Peyronie disease

Peyronie disease is a condition that occurs in a small percentage of men who've had prostatectomy surgery. It results from fibrous scar tissue that develops on the penis and causes curved erections that can be painful.

This condition is often not recognized by men until they seek treatment for erectile dysfunction. The condition may worsen erectile dysfunction, and the curvature can be severe enough that it prevents normal intercourse.

The objective of treatment is to improve the curvature of the penis and to make it so that normal intercourse is possible. Treatment for the condition may include penile traction therapy, oral or injected medications or surgery. The treatment your doctor recommends will depend in part on whether your disease is in an active or chronic stage.

Injected medications are generally more effective than oral medications. You'll likely receive multiple injections over several months. Traction therapy is typically most effective in the early phase of Peyronie disease. It's the only treatment shown to improve penile length. Traction therapy may also be used in the chronic phase of the disease, combined with other treatments or after surgery to help achieve a better outcome. Surgery is generally considered if the deformity of

the penis is severe, significantly bothersome or prevents you from having sex.

MANAGING BOWEL DISORDERS

Some men who receive radiation therapy for prostate cancer experience a variety of gastrointestinal complications. These may include blood in the stool, cramps, rectal irritation and discharge, diarrhea, and a feeling of urinary urgency. Generally, these complications are annoying and worrisome but temporary.

External beam radiation is very accurate in targeting prostate cancer, but your rectum may also receive some of the radiation. The most common side effect is rectal irritation. This irritation should lessen once treatment is completed, but sometimes it can persist. Injury from radiation that requires surgical repair is rare.

Prostate surgery can also cause rectal injury, but this is rare. If there is any type of damage, it's usually repaired during the surgery and doesn't cause lasting effects.

The bowel problems may continue for several months after prostate treatment. Most will improve on their own.

Blood in the stool

Radiation therapy can injure the lining of the rectum. One result is the abnormal growth of tiny blood vessels (capillaries) within the outermost lining of the rectum.

These capillaries have thin, fragile walls that tear or rupture easily, resulting in bleeding. Sometimes, rectal bleeding can continue for years after treatment.

Treatment depends on the severity of the bleeding. Often, the first step is to monitor the bleeding to see if you're passing only small amounts of blood. If the bleeding is moderate to heavy, your doctor may prescribe stool softeners or medicated enemas to reduce pressure on your rectal lining as stool passes. For severe cases, laser therapy can often destroy or seal off the blood vessels causing the bleeding.

Diarrhea

Diarrhea may result from radiation therapy, but this usually occurs only when it's necessary to treat the entire pelvic region. Signs and symptoms include frequent, loose, watery stools; abdominal cramps and pain; and bloating. Generally, these effects are temporary. Over-the-counter antidiarrheal medications may help reduce your symptoms.

Diarrhea can cause the loss of significant amounts of water and salts from your body. To prevent dehydration during episodes of diarrhea, drink at least eight glasses of clear liquids daily, including water or clear sodas. Avoid dairy products, caffeine, and fatty or highly seasoned foods, which can prolong diarrhea. Warning signs of dehydration include excessive thirst, dry mouth, weakness, dark-colored urine, and little or no urination.

Constipation

Medications used to treat prostate cancer may reduce the normal activity of your bowels and delay bowel movements. When this happens, fecal material becomes packed and hard, producing cramps and constipation. Signs and symptoms of constipation include passing hard stools, straining frequently during bowel movements, and bloating and abdominal discomfort.

Fortunately, you may be able to relieve constipation by following a regular eating schedule that includes high-fiber foods, such as whole-grain cereals and breads, fresh vegetables, and fresh fruits. To avoid possible discomfort caused by gas, add these foods to your diet gradually. Daily exercise and drinking plenty of fluids also will help prevent constipation.

If these measures don't help, several types of laxatives exist. Each works somewhat differently to make it easier to have a bowel movement. The following products are available over the counter:
- **Fiber supplements.** Fiber supplements add bulk to your stool. Bulky stools are softer and easier to pass. Fiber supplements include psyllium (Metamucil, Konsyl, others), calcium polycarbophil (FiberCon, Equalactin, others) and methylcellulose (Citrucel).
- **Stimulants.** Stimulants including bisacodyl (Correctol, Dulcolax, others) and sennosides (Senokot, ex-lax, Perdiem) cause your intestines to contract.
- **Osmotics.** Osmotic laxatives help stool move through the colon by increasing

secretion of fluid from the intestines and helping stimulate bowel movements. Examples include oral magnesium hydroxide (Phillips' Milk of Magnesia, Dulcolax Milk of Magnesia, others), magnesium citrate, lactulose (Cholac, Constilac, others), polyethylene glycol (Miralax, GlycoLax).

- **Lubricants.** Lubricants such as mineral oil enable stool to move through your colon more easily.
- **Stool softeners.** Stool softeners such as docusate sodium (Colace) and docusate calcium (Surfak) moisten the stool by drawing water from the intestines.
- **Enemas and suppositories.** Tap water enemas with or without soapsuds can be useful to soften stool and produce a bowel movement. Glycerin or bisacodyl suppositories also aid in moving stool out of the body by providing lubrication and stimulation.

If over-the-counter products don't help your chronic constipation, talk to your doctor who may recommend a prescription medication.

ANSWERS TO YOUR QUESTIONS

How long should I expect to wear absorbent underwear after treatment for prostate cancer?

The length of time varies, but it's common for men to wear absorbent products for 1 to 4 months after treatment.

What's the difference between impotence and erectile dysfunction?

The terms are often used interchangeably, but they aren't exactly the same. Impotence means that your penis is unable to become firm (erect) or stay firm long enough to have sexual intercourse. Erectile dysfunction includes impotence plus other abnormalities, such as a prolonged erection or abnormal curvature of the penis.

If I have good erections before treatment, does that increase the chance I'll be able to have normal erections afterward?

Yes. Younger, healthier men experiencing strong erections are far more likely to continue normal erections after treatment than are older men or men already having erectile problems.

Are treatments for incontinence and erectile dysfunction covered by Medicare?

Most are. However, Medicare may not pay the entire cost, especially for medications. You may have to pay a portion of the cost yourself.

10

Getting on with life

Receiving a diagnosis of prostate cancer may have been one of the most difficult challenges you've faced. The diagnosis may have consumed your thoughts and actions, and your treatment and recovery may have produced many long-lasting changes to your daily routine, relationships and outlook on life.

At first, you may have struggled to retain a sense of normalcy in your life. You may have experienced a wide range of emotions, including disbelief, anger, anxiety, emptiness and depression. In addition, side effects from your treatment and recovery may have been difficult to accept and manage.

Now, you may be wondering what more the future has in store for you: What will your quality of life be like? Can you

expect to see improvements? Will you be able to accomplish all you hoped in life?

Although prostate cancer remains a serious illness, it's no longer considered an inevitable death sentence. Knowledge of the cancer — its effect on your body, how to detect it and how best to treat it — has come a long way. Increasingly, prostate cancer is becoming a tale of survivorship. Life with and after prostate cancer is not only possible but also can be fulfilling.

MEDICAL VISITS

Some men dread visiting their doctors after treatment of prostate cancer. This is natural. A routine doctor visit is probably how they first became aware of this life-changing development. So, it's understandable that follow-up care can cause feelings of anxiety, stress and worry for fear of a recurrence. If this is you, try to balance your anxiety with positive thoughts. Knowing what to expect with your future care can also be helpful in calming your anxieties.

Talk to your doctor and ask questions regarding how frequently you'll need checkups and what tests you'll receive. At first, you may need to see your doctor every 3 months. Eventually, your visits may be just once or twice a year. In addition to a physical exam, some check-ups may include X-rays or tests, such as a prostate-specific antigen (PSA) test, to make sure the cancer hasn't returned — or that it hasn't spread, if you're living with advanced cancer.

EMOTIONAL TOLL

Prostate cancer can produce a roller coaster of emotions but know that there's no right way to feel or act if you have cancer. Feelings are simply feelings — they aren't right or wrong. It's what you do with those feelings — recognizing and dealing with them instead of bottling them up — that's the most important.

TALKING TO YOUR DOCTOR

Most men have questions about what to expect after treatment for prostate cancer. Here are 10 questions you might ask your doctor. You likely have others to add to this list:

1. How long will it take for me to get better and feel more like myself?
2. What kind of care should I expect after treatment?
3. What doctor(s) will I see for my follow-up care? How often?
4. What tests do I need after my treatment is over? How often will I have the tests?
5. What long-term health issues can I expect as a result of my cancer and its treatment?
6. What symptoms should I tell you about?
7. Who do I call if I develop these symptoms?
8. What's the chance that my cancer will return?
9. What can I do to be as healthy as possible?
10. Is there a support group that you would recommend?

Based on information from the National Cancer Institute, 2019.

What to expect

Certain feelings and emotions seem to be more common than others among men coping with prostate cancer. You may experience all of them, just a few of them or none.

Anxiety

The distress caused by your diagnosis and treatment or just living with cancer can lead to anxiety. You may be anxious about tests and procedures, changes to your body, loss of control, a cancer recurrence or death. These feelings are normal.

If you experience side effects from your treatment, such as incontinence or erectile dysfunction, talking about them may embarrass you. Such side effects can also undermine your self-confidence. You may find yourself withdrawing from social settings because you're afraid of embarrassing yourself.

Common signs and symptoms of anxiety include:
- Intense fear or worry.
- Restlessness or irritability.
- Trouble sleeping or waking up feeling wired.
- Fatigue or loss of energy.
- Impaired concentration.
- A rapid pulse, shortness of breath and trembling.

A good relationship with your doctor can help you deal with some of the fears and concerns that fuel anxiety. Family and friends also can provide support by helping reduce the amount of stress in your life.

Typically, anxiety tends to dissipate as you adjust to the changes you're going through. But sometimes the feelings persist. Fortunately, anxiety is treatable, and addressing it promptly can enhance your well-being and make your cancer less worrisome.

Depression

When you first learn that you have cancer, you may become discouraged and pessimistic about your future or about having to live with potential side effects of the cancer, such as erectile dysfunction or incontinence. Negative feelings can take time to work through, but they usually become more manageable over weeks or months.

Among some people, however, such feelings deepen and linger. Grief and discouragement can evolve into major depression. This can precipitate a downward spiral that makes you more miserable. Because you're depressed, you don't put effort into coping with your daily problems. And when the problems worsen, so does your depression.

Major depression is characterized by a change in mood that lasts for more than 2 weeks. Signs and symptoms of depression include:
- Persistent anger or sadness.
- Irritability or feelings of anxiety.
- Lack of interest in most activities.
- Fatigue or loss of energy.

FEAR OF RECURRENCE

One of the most common fears among prostate cancer survivors is that the cancer will come back. While it's true that cancer can recur after treatment, it's also true that many men never experience a recurrence.

We live in a world that emphasizes facts and knowledge. Despite certain clues about the general outcome of prostate cancer and cancer treatment, it's impossible to foretell the future. Therefore, you and your doctor must learn to live with some degree of uncertainty.

Some anxiety about recurrence is healthy — for example, it prompts you to respond to unusual signs and symptoms. Being continuously anxious, however, can rob you of time that might be spent in a more worthwhile manner, such as focusing on work or family or simply enjoying life.

If you find that fears of recurrence are taking a toll, discuss them with your doctor. He or she can recommend programs or stress-reduction techniques that help you move through and beyond the fears so that you can enjoy each day to the fullest.

- Noticeable changes in appetite and sleep patterns.
- Feelings of helplessness, hopelessness, worthlessness or guilt.
- Continuous negative thinking.
- Impaired concentration.
- Recurrent thoughts of death or suicide.

Depression is a serious health problem — it's not a passing phase that simply goes away on its own. When left untreated, symptoms of depression tend to worsen.

Depression generally isn't something you can handle on your own. It should be professionally treated. Learn to recognize the symptoms of depression and consult your doctor if you feel that you could be developing depression.

Similar to anxiety, treatment for depression usually involves a combination of medications and therapy sessions with a psychiatrist or mental health professional. Most people who seek treatment show improvement within a matter of weeks.

If you're in the midst of active cancer treatment, getting a handle on depression can help you better cope with your treatment and any potential side effects. Treatment of depression also can improve relationships with family and friends and may help you to be more productive.

Wrestling with heavy emotions, such as anxiety and depression, can contribute to fatigue. Relaxation helps to relieve the stress and anxiety that make it difficult to concentrate and recuperate. Talk to your doctor or a member of your health care team about stress-reduction techniques, and which ones might work best for you.

Deep breathing. With deep breathing, you take deep, evenly paced breaths using the muscle under your rib cage (diaphragm). Breathing from your diaphragm is more relaxing than is breathing from your chest. It exchanges more carbon dioxide for oxygen, giving you more energy. To practice deep breathing, take a deep breath of air, pause, slowly exhale, and then pause before repeating. Deep breathing produces natural painkillers (endorphins) within your body, and it reduces the amount of stress chemicals in your brain and relaxes your muscles.

Progressive muscle relaxation. This technique involves tightening and relaxing a series of muscles one at a time. Start either at your head or your feet, then move in sequence to the other end of your body. First, raise the tension level in a group of muscles, such as your neck muscles, by tightening the muscles and then slowly relaxing them. Concentrate on letting the tension go in each muscle. Then move on to the next muscle group. In addition to helping relax tense muscles, progressive muscle relaxation helps relieve anxiety and stress.

Word repetition. Choose a word or phrase that's a cue for you to relax, and then repeat it. While repeating the word or phrase, you might close your eyes. Try to breathe deeply and slowly and think of something that gives you pleasant sensations of warmth and heaviness.

Guided imagery. Close your eyes and use all of your senses to imagine a scene that brings you feelings of peace. For instance, imagine lying on a beach. Picture the beautiful blue sky, smell the salt water, hear the waves, and feel the warm breeze on your skin. The messages your brain receives help calm and relax you.

Other commonly used relaxation techniques include massage, meditation, yoga and tai chi. Whichever technique you choose, try to practice regularly to reap the benefits.

Sense of loss

If you undergo surgery to remove your prostate gland, you may feel an emptiness that's hard to describe — especially if the surgery causes erectile dysfunction. Cancer treatment may also reduce or eliminate the production of male hormones, mainly testosterone, which can also affect how you respond to sexual stimulation.

Because of these changes, you might get the feeling that you're somehow less of a man — just as some women may feel they're less feminine after breast removal. Fortunately, as discussed in Chapter 9, treatments for erectile dysfunction are available that can help ease these concerns.

What you can do

As you learn to cope with changes in your life, your emotions should become more manageable. Many people are surprised to discover reserves of strength they never thought they had. You may still have times when you struggle with feelings of anxiety or discouragement, even years later. This is normal. What's important is that the balance of your emotions leans to the positive side. The following strategies may help you cope with some of the residual effects of prostate cancer.

Be prepared

Educating yourself about prostate cancer, its treatment and follow-up care can help you feel more in control of your life. Write down questions and concerns and bring them with you to doctor visits. Often, the fewer surprises you face, the more quickly you can adapt. But don't let your quest for knowledge become an obsession, which may cause you more stress or to second-guess your doctor.

Maintain a normal routine

Don't let the cancer or the side effects of treatment control your life. Try to maintain a semblance of your former lifestyle and daily routine. You'll do better if you can engage in activities that give you a sense of purpose, fulfillment and meaning — return to work, take a trip or join a family outing. If you have health limitations, give yourself permission to start slowly and gradually build your level of endurance.

Build a positive support system

Your mind and body aren't separate entities. The better you feel emotionally, the better able you'll be to physically cope with cancer and recovery. Surrounding yourself with caring people who support you will boost your spirits and give you confidence.

Take care of your body

Get enough sleep, eat a healthy diet and exercise regularly, as you're able. Exercise helps release muscle tension, reduce stress, reduce signs and symptoms of depression, improve a negative mood, increase self-esteem and improve your quality of life. Learn more about diet and exercise in this chapter and in Chapter 11.

Maintain sexual intimacy

Your natural reaction to erectile dysfunction may be to avoid all sexual contact. Resist this course of action — there are many ways to express your sexuality.

Touching, holding, hugging and caressing may become far more important to you and your partner. In fact, the closeness you develop in these actions can produce greater sexual intimacy than you had before.

Look for the silver lining

Cancer doesn't have to be all negative — good can come out of your experience.

SPIRITUALITY AND HEALING

Spirituality — in its broadest sense — describes a powerful resource that resides in the human spirit and soul. For some people, spirituality emerges in the form of religious practice. You may also experience spirituality through music, art, nature or solitude.

Numerous studies have attempted to measure the effect of spirituality on illness and recovery. Many researchers believe that people who consider themselves to be spiritual enjoy better health, live longer, recover from illness more quickly and with fewer complications, have less depression and chemical addiction, have lower blood pressure and cope better with serious disease, including cancer.

No one knows exactly how spirituality affects health. Some experts attribute the healing effect to hope, which is known to benefit your immune system. Others liken spiritual acts and beliefs to meditation, which decreases muscle tension and can lower your heart rate. Still others point to the social connectedness that spirituality often provides.

Practicing spirituality may speed healing and improve your health, but keep in mind that spirituality isn't a cure. There aren't any studies that have found that prayer, art, music or nature actually cure health problems. Think of spirituality as a helpful healing force — as a supplement to, but not a substitute for, traditional medical care.

Confrontation with cancer may lead you to grow, both emotionally and spiritually. It may also help you identify what really matters to you, settle long-standing disputes and spend more time with the people who are important to you.

REGAINING YOUR STRENGTH

Fatigue is one of the most common side effects of prostate cancer. It may be associated with the physical effects of treatment and recovery. It also can stem from the emotional toll that cancer can take.

Cancer-related fatigue may result from:
- Stress, anxiety and depression.
- Sleep disturbances.
- Surgery or radiation therapy.
- Metabolic abnormalities related to the cancer or its treatment.
- Low red blood cell count (anemia) from the cancer or its treatment.

Other factors that may contribute to fatigue include certain medications, poor nutrition and a lack of physical activity.

For someone who hasn't experienced cancer-related fatigue, it may be difficult to grasp what it's like. Everyone knows what it feels like to run out of steam after a hectic day, but a little rest usually helps you bounce back. Cancer-related fatigue is more pervasive. Some rest may not make it better.

If you're experiencing fatigue, talk to a member of your health care team for strategies to help conserve your energy.

Self-care for fatigue

Ignoring exhaustion and pushing yourself too hard can make your fatigue worse. At the same time, additional rest or sleep doesn't always cure fatigue. Find help from your social network. It's important to accept that you can't do it all. Call on friends and family to help with chores and errands.

Other steps that may help reduce fatigue include:
- Plan activities for times when you have the most energy.
- Look for ways to conserve energy. For example, sit on a stool when you're in the workshop or kitchen.
- Delegate chores that wear you out. But don't use your illness as an excuse to avoid all chores — some physical activity is good.
- Pace yourself and take short naps or rest breaks when you need them.
- Get some exercise each day. Moderate exercise after cancer treatment is strongly recommended.
- Eat a good breakfast to prepare your body for the day's demands and refuel every 3 or 4 hours.
- Make sure you're drinking enough fluids to avoid dehydration, which can contribute to fatigue.
- Talk to your doctor if fatigue remains a problem.

To overcome fatigue, it's also important to get a good night's sleep. Here are some suggestions that may help you sleep better:
- Get in the habit of going to bed and waking up at about the same times.

This helps your body establish a regular sleep cycle.

- Develop a relaxing routine before bed, such as bathing, reading or listening to music. This signals your body to prepare for sleep.
- Avoid foods and beverages that can disrupt sleep. Anything with caffeine, such as coffee or chocolate, can make it more difficult to fall asleep. Alcoholic drinks may help you fall asleep, but they can disrupt deep-sleep patterns.
- Drink fewer beverages before bed so you don't have to get up during the night to go to the bathroom.
- Get at least 30 minutes of physical activity if you can — preferably 5 to 6 hours before you go to bed — and keep active during the day, without overdoing it.
- Keep your bedroom temperature comfortable and use a fan or ambient sound to block out noise.

EATING BETTER TO FEEL BETTER

Food provides the fuel that allows your body to maintain its strength and function best. A nutritious diet is especially important when your body is undergoing the rigors of cancer treatment and recovery.

Some therapies used to treat prostate cancer, especially chemotherapy, may cause nausea and vomiting. You also may find that food doesn't taste the way it used to, making it less appealing. Side effects such as depression and stress associated with cancer treatment also can affect your appetite.

During treatment or recovery, your diet may differ from your normal diet. Focus on calories and protein:

- **Calories.** If you don't eat enough food or the right kinds of food, your body resorts to using nutrients stored in cells. Drawing on these reserves may weaken your natural defenses against infection. To prevent this, try to eat high-calorie foods that promote energy. Maintaining your weight is a helpful sign that you're eating enough.
- **Protein.** Include plenty of protein in your diet because it gives you strength and helps repair body tissues.

Nutritional drinks

Nutritional drinks can be used as meal substitutes if you don't feel like eating. You can also drink them between meals in order to increase calories, protein and other nutrients. Because the drinks need no refrigeration, you may carry them with you and have them whenever you feel hungry or thirsty.

Nutritional drinks, commonly available in liquid or powder form, are sold under brand names such as Ensure, Sustacal, Boost and Carnation Breakfast Essentials. The drinks are high in calories and protein and contain extra vitamins and minerals.

Some people find nutritional products difficult to drink because they don't care for the flavor or texture. If this is true for you, try this simple recipe and see if it improves the product's appeal: Combine one can of a liquid drink with a piece of fruit or a scoop of ice cream. Blend the mixture in a blender and serve over ice.

Stimulating your appetite

The following tips may help improve your diet and stimulate your appetite:

- **Eat lightly and frequently.** Eating smaller meals or munching on healthy snacks throughout the day may work better than three large meals.
- **Choose foods that look and smell good to you.** Some cancer treatments can change your sense of taste and smell. If red meat becomes unappetizing, for example, eat chicken, fish or another protein.
- **Be willing to try new foods.** You may find that some foods you used to love now don't taste as good. On the other hand, foods you used to avoid may now be more appealing. Give them a try.
- **Prepare and freeze favorite meals ahead of time.** This way you don't have to cook on days when you don't feel up to it. Instead, you just need to thaw and heat the meal.
- **Drink less with meals.** Try to limit beverages at mealtimes because they

CURBING NAUSEA AND DIARRHEA

Radiation, certain medications and anxiety all may contribute to nausea and diarrhea. Here are some suggestions that may help you combat these conditions:

Nausea

- Eat something dry, such as a piece of toast or saltine crackers, right after you wake up in the morning.
- Eat mild-flavored foods low in fat, such as cereals, rice, noodles, baked potatoes, lean meats, fruits and vegetables.
- Eat cold foods or foods at room temperature. They may be more appealing because they produce less odor than hot foods.
- Avoid foods more likely to trigger nausea, such as overly sweet, fried, spicy or fatty foods.
- Sit up for 10 to 20 minutes after you eat and let your food settle.

Diarrhea

- Drink plenty of clear fluids.
- Eat food in small amounts throughout the day instead of three large meals.
- Avoid greasy foods, foods with skins or seeds, and gas-forming vegetables, such as broccoli, cabbage and cauliflower.
- Consume foods and beverages that contain potassium and sodium — two minerals often lost during diarrhea. High-sodium liquids include bouillon and broth. Foods and beverages high in potassium include bananas, peach or apricot nectar, and boiled or mashed potatoes. Sports drinks also contain high levels of both sodium and potassium.

can make you feel full when you're not. Instead, save them for the end of the meal.

- **Change the atmosphere.** Eating in a different setting may stimulate your appetite. Invite a friend over, play music, light some candles, or watch a favorite television program.

If you still have trouble eating a few weeks after your treatment, talk to your health care team for advice. A registered dietitian can devise an eating plan that's suited to your tastes and nutritional needs.

CONTINUING TO WORK

Having cancer doesn't mean that your career is finished, or you'll never again be able to pull your weight on the job. In fact, the vast majority of people with cancer do return to work. Surveys show that people who've been treated for cancer can be just as productive as other workers, and no more likely to take sick days.

Your job may be an important part of your life, contributing to your personal fulfillment, self-image, income, enjoyment and sense of community. A job can also be therapeutic in times of illness, providing a welcome distraction from your cancer. Many men with prostate cancer find that getting back to work helps them regain a sense of normalcy in their lives.

At first, you may need to make a few adjustments. Work can be exhausting if you try to do too much too soon. But eventually you should be able to resume your typical routine.

Under the Americans with Disabilities Act, your employer is required by law to make reasonable accommodations that enable you to work while you're undergoing treatment and recuperating. However, these laws may not apply to certain organizations, such as employers with fewer than 15 employees.

Talk to your doctor about how to ease back into a work schedule. And discuss with your employer possible accommodations, including flexible work hours, working from home or moving your workstation to a more convenient location. Initially, you may need to take sick leave, vacation with pay or unpaid leave.

COMMUNICATING WITH OTHERS

Cancer has a way of stifling communication at a time when a hug, a thoughtful word or a personal conversation can be helpful. Family members may have difficulty coming to grips with your illness, which may prevent them from talking about the important issues. Well-meaning friends — not knowing what to say or do, and not wanting to upset you — may avoid conversations about your health or may avoid you.

During this time, you also may not feel comfortable answering questions or sharing your feelings.

A period of adjustment may be necessary for everyone involved.

Accept that emotional timetables are different for everyone. You may want to talk about important issues related to your illness before some of your family and friends are ready. If they're not ready to talk, give them more time to adjust.

If a loved one is ready to talk before you are, postpone the discussion without hurting the person's feelings. Place responsibility on yourself by saying, "I know we need to make some decisions, but I really need a little more time."

Not all families are open and sharing. You or a family member may find it difficult to discuss feelings openly. Sometimes, it's easier to talk to someone outside your circle of friends, such as a counselor, support group or a cancer survivor.

For some of your family and friends, you may need to be the person who makes the first step, even if you think it should be the other way around. Recall people in your past who were ill and how hard it may have been for you to think of what to say or do to help them.

As you reach out, find ways to put family and friends at ease. Inquire about what they have going on or what projects they're working on. Invite someone who's not a great talker to help you with a task.

Many times, family and friends are looking for opportunities to help, and they're just waiting for an invitation from you to offer their support. Most people are grateful to have a chance to show you, in practical ways, that they care.

FINDING SUPPORT

In the days and weeks after completing cancer treatment, you may feel as if you're suddenly alone in the world. Friends and family can help fill the void, but sometimes only fellow cancer survivors — people who've been there — can provide you the knowledge and understanding you need.

Cancer support groups bring together people who've had cancer. Participants talk about their personal experiences and feelings, they listen to the concerns of others, and they discuss the challenges of life after cancer. Not everyone needs a support group. Having family and friends may be all the support you need. But some people find it helpful to interact with others outside their immediate circles.

In general, support groups fall into two main categories — those led by health care professionals, such as a psychologist or nurse, and those led by group members, cancer survivors themselves. Some are structured and educational. Others emphasize emotional support and shared experiences. Some focus on a specific kind of cancer, while others are broader and include people with all types of cancer.

No matter how the support group is set up, the goal should be the same. Attending the meetings should be beneficial and comforting, helping you to cope and live better with cancer. If you find the experience awkward or uncomfortable, trust your instincts and stop attending the meetings. Some groups that aren't carefully monitored can become a place to share only negative feelings. This environment may leave you depressed and add to your frustration.

Benefits

The key to a successful experience with a support group is finding one that matches your needs and personality. The benefits you may receive include:
- **Sense of belonging.** A special camaraderie often forms among group members. When you feel accepted in the group, you may also become more accepting of yourself.
- **Understanding.** Support group members have firsthand knowledge of what you're experiencing without you having to explain it to them. You may express feelings without fear that you'll be misunderstood.
- **Exchange of advice.** When group members talk, you know they speak from experience. They can describe coping techniques that have worked for them and those that haven't helped.
- **Friendship.** Group members can bring some joy into your life as well as practical support — a listening ear when you need to talk, a chauffeur when you could use a relaxing drive, or a companion to exercise with.

As a cautionary note, support groups can also include people offering opinions that aren't well founded, and even potentially harmful. It's always best to consider any advice in relation to information you've received from your health care team.

Consult your doctor or another team member before taking any action.

Support groups also are available online. Online support groups are convenient; however, similar to in-person groups, be careful about the reliability of the information you receive. Avoid groups that promise a cure or claim to be a substitute for medical treatment. Look

IS A SUPPORT GROUP RIGHT FOR YOU?

If you're thinking of joining a support group, here are a few questions to ask about the group to see if it's a good fit:
- How large is the group?
- Who attends (survivors or family members, types of cancer, age range)?
- How often does the group meet?
- How long are the meetings?
- How long has the group been together?
- Who leads the meetings — a professional or a survivor?
- What's the format of the meetings?
- Is the main purpose to share feelings, or offer and share advice?
- If I go, can I just sit and listen?

Additionally, you may want to ask yourself:
- Am I comfortable talking about personal issues?
- What do I hope to gain by joining a support group?

Based on information from the National Cancer Institute, 2019.

for groups affiliated with a reputable organization or hosted by medical experts.

It's also important to know that there are support groups that are geared toward helping spouses or other loved ones who are living with or caring for an individual experiencing cancer.

Finding a support group

The support group you choose may depend largely on what's available in your local community. To find a local support group:
- Ask your doctor or a member of your health care team for assistance.
- Look for a listing of support groups in your area online or in local publications.
- Contact community centers, libraries or religious organizations.
- Ask others you know who've had cancer if they know of a group.
- Contact a national cancer organization such as the American Cancer Society or ZERO: The End of Prostate Cancer (see pages 220-221).

ANSWERS TO YOUR QUESTIONS

What if, months after treatment, a PSA test produces an elevated reading? Does this mean the cancer is back?

If you still have your prostate gland, an elevated PSA level may occur for reasons other than cancer, or it may be an indication the cancer has returned or is progressing. Elevated PSA levels after removal of the prostate usually indicate that cancer is present.

How long will it take after surgery before I can exercise and take part in sporting activities again?

Fatigue can linger for 3 to 6 months after surgery. Your ability to participate also depends on the activity and your physical condition before surgery. Somewhere between 6 weeks and 2 months after surgery you may be able to jog, golf, swim or play tennis at a leisurely pace. It may be many months, however, before you can ride a bicycle or a horse. A bicycle seat or a saddle places pressure on the lower pelvis, the location of the surgery.

What's a living will?

A living will, also known as an advance directive, is a legal document that states your wishes about your medical care in case of a terminal illness. For example, it states whether you want to be placed on a breathing device (ventilator) or have a feeding tube. If you choose to prepare a living will, it's important that people in charge of your care, such as your doctor and a family member, receive copies.

Does the fear that the cancer will return ever go away?

Some people are able to get past this fear. Others aren't. But in most cases, the fear wanes as the months and years pass. No one expects you to forget that you've had cancer. But your fears will become few and far between as you fill your mind and time with other thoughts and activities.

4

Prostate health

11

Can you prevent prostate disease?

Changes that occur in the prostate gland are likely the result of many factors, including genetics, environment and physical health, in addition to age. Although prostate disorders are a common problem for many men, that doesn't mean they're inevitable.

The combination of factors that may trigger prostate problems varies from person to person. There's no formula guaranteeing that you won't get prostate disease, but there are definite steps that you can take to reduce your risk, or possibly slow disease progression.

Three important steps may help keep your prostate healthy. They're also excellent steps for maintaining overall health. You may already have been practicing them for many years:

- Eat well.
- Keep physically active.
- See your doctor regularly.

How much benefit you'll receive by following these steps is unknown. While there are indications good health practices may benefit the prostate gland, there's no way to be certain if they actually prevent prostate inflammation, enlargement or cancer. However, these steps will make your body stronger and keep you healthier.

If you haven't made a point to incorporate healthy behaviors into your lifestyle, there's no time like the present to start. Even small changes — maybe an extra serving of vegetables each day or an added walk or jog a few times a week — can make an impact.

POTENTIAL CANCER-FIGHTING FOODS

Researchers continue to investigate certain foods and beverages to see if they might help reduce the risk of prostate disease, especially cancer. Studies to this point have been inconclusive. Regardless, these foods are part of a healthy diet, and you should have few concerns about including them in meals.

Antioxidant-rich foods

Antioxidants are substances that protect your body's cells from the effects of free radicals — unstable molecules that turn toxic when they're produced in overabundance. Damage from free radicals may cause cancer. Antioxidants help stabilize the molecules, reducing their potential for damage.

Studies so far have been inconclusive and haven't established a direct link between the antioxidant properties of certain foods and the prevention of disease. Nevertheless, increasing your intake of foods rich in antioxidants appears to improve nutrition and enhance your overall health.

Antioxidants are found in many vegetables and fruits, especially those with intense color — red, purple, blue, orange and yellow. Other sources of antioxidants are nuts and grains, and some meats, poultry and fish.

Tomatoes and tomato products contain lycopene, an antioxidant that gives the fruit its red color. Studies have shown that there are more antioxidants in cooked tomato products — soups as well as sauces used in spaghetti and pizza — than in raw products such as fresh tomatoes or tomato juice. On the other hand, broccoli provides more antioxidants in its raw form than in its cooked form.

While antioxidant-rich foods are a great idea, it's important not to overdo your intake, to avoid consuming excessive amounts of antioxidants. Consumption of antioxidants beyond your body's ability to use them could lead to increased production of free radicals. This is a big reason why it's probably best to get your antioxidants from food rather than from supplements.

Soy

The soybean is part of the family of beans, peas and lentils called legumes. It's native to northern China and now commonly grown in the United States. Fermentation techniques allow soy to be prepared in a variety of forms, including tempeh, miso, tofu and tamari (soy) sauce.

Active compounds in soy called isoflavones appear to help keep the sex hormones testosterone and estrogen in check. Because prostate cancer cells feed off testosterone, researchers theorize that reducing the hormone's effect may lower your risk of cancer. A recent review found that men who ate large amounts of nonfermented soy, such as tofu, had a lower risk of prostate cancer. However, the same reduction in risk wasn't found

SOURCES OF SOY

Soy isn't a common ingredient in foods, but you can find items containing soy in well-stocked grocery and health food stores.

Dried soybeans. Soak the beans overnight and then cook to soften. You may also find precooked products. Add the beans to your favorite recipes, including soups, chilies, stir-fries or salads.

Tofu. Its neutral taste and spongy texture make it ideal for absorbing other flavors. Substitute it in place of meat for a main course.

Tempeh and miso. Tempeh is available in a thin cake, and miso is a paste. Both can be used in soups and salads or as a meat substitute.

Textured soy protein (TSP). Available in the frozen food section, TSP is found in soy burgers and can be used in casseroles or foods such as tacos.

Soy milk. Use it in recipes or on cereal.

Soy flour. It can be substituted for a portion of all-purpose flour in many baked goods. You can also substitute 1 tablespoon of soy flour with 1 to 2 tablespoons of water for each egg in recipes for baked goods.

when consuming fermented products, such as miso.

In Asia, where soy is a food staple, certain types of cancers, including prostate and breast cancers, are less common. But it's uncertain whether this benefit is due to soy or some other aspect of the Asian lifestyle — for example, the Asian diet is much lower in fat than the typical American diet.

Soy also provides fiber, vitamins and minerals, and is a great source of dietary protein because it doesn't contain all the fat and cholesterol found in meat. Claims that soy can reduce cholesterol levels are unconfirmed.

Green tea

Green tea contains polyphenols — compounds with strong antioxidant qualities. Some studies involving green tea have shown a short-term decrease in prostate-specific antigen (PSA) levels or lower risk of prostate cancer, particularly in men at

VITAMINS AND MINERALS

Research exploring the role of vitamins and minerals in preventing prostate cancer is inconclusive. Past studies suggested vitamins and minerals may reduce risk, but other research indicates no such benefit. Several studies have focused on whether vitamins such as D, E and the mineral selenium may help prevent prostate disease.

The Selenium and Vitamin E Cancer Prevention Trial (SELECT) — a major study funded in part by the National Cancer Institute — was halted when it was determined that vitamin E and selenium, taken alone or together, showed no evidence of preventing prostate cancer, and in some cases was associated with an increased risk. The SELECT study suggested that men with prostate cancer should not take selenium supplements.

Most doctors don't recommend taking individual supplements for the sole purpose of reducing the risk of prostate disease. Not enough is known about their role in preventing disease, or at what dosage they should be taken. High doses of some vitamins and minerals may be toxic.

If you believe your diet isn't giving you all the nutrients you need, there's little harm in taking a daily multivitamin. But it's best to get your vitamins and minerals from whole foods so you can benefit from the other nutrients food provides. Try not to exceed the recommended dietary allowances for vitamins and minerals.

high risk for the disease. Other studies, however, have not.

Clinical trials to date typically have involved a small number of participants, and it's not known whether the decline in PSA levels or reduction in disease were from the green tea or other lifestyle factors. In those studies where a benefit was seen, a large daily consumption of green tea was required to register any benefits.

More research is needed to determine whether green tea can prevent or treat prostate cancer, but the tea does appear to have some medicinal qualities and doesn't cause significant complications. Studies on green tea extract are ongoing.

Cruciferous vegetables

Cruciferous vegetables include bok choy, broccoli, Brussels sprouts, cabbage,

DAIRY PRODUCTS AND PROSTATE CANCER

Debate continues regarding a link between milk consumption and prostate cancer. Some studies indicate that a high calcium intake — primarily from dairy products — may increase prostate cancer risk. Researchers theorize that the extra calcium suppresses a hormone believed to protect against cancer.

A 2021 review found that increased milk consumption was associated with an increased risk of developing prostate cancer in many of the studies it analyzed. But other studies didn't find this link, and in some of the research, calcium consumption was well above the recommended daily intake.

So, it's important to keep this caveat in mind: Dairy products, dietary calcium and prostate cancer may be related to other factors. More research is needed to determine whether calcium or fat or some other component in dairy products is responsible for the increased risk. If you're at high risk of prostate cancer, talk with your health care provider about whether you should be limiting dairy products and about healthy calcium alternatives.

Calcium supplements and nondairy calcium sources, such as tofu and kale, aren't associated with increased prostate cancer risk.

cauliflower, collards, kale, rutabagas and turnips. Studies haven't established a link between dietary intake and cancer prevention. However, some research suggests eating cruciferous vegetables may reduce the incidence of prostate cancer.

Garlic

In regions of the world where people eat a lot of garlic, there tends to be less prostate cancer. However, study results have been inconclusive, and some studies have used multi-ingredient products, making it difficult to know if garlic alone is responsible for the benefit. Regardless, you shouldn't have any worries about including garlic in your diet to enhance the flavor of foods.

A HEALTHY DIET

The relationship between diet and health is very powerful. The food you eat each day and the nutrients that food provides can prevent several medical conditions, including obesity, cardiovascular disease, diabetes and cancer, to name a few.

Research indicates that diets high in vegetables and fruits, whole grains, nuts, and lean proteins can protect against many health problems, including cancer. Controlling fat and calories is important to good health, and it may be especially important in preventing prostate cancer.

Several studies have suggested a possible link between diets high in calories and fat

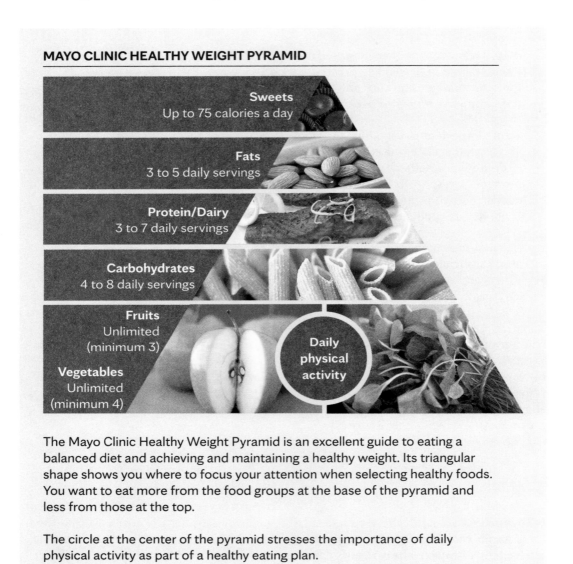

MAYO CLINIC HEALTHY WEIGHT PYRAMID

Sweets
Up to 75 calories a day

Fats
3 to 5 daily servings

Protein/Dairy
3 to 7 daily servings

Carbohydrates
4 to 8 daily servings

Fruits
Unlimited
(minimum 3)

Daily physical activity

Vegetables
Unlimited
(minimum 4)

The Mayo Clinic Healthy Weight Pyramid is an excellent guide to eating a balanced diet and achieving and maintaining a healthy weight. Its triangular shape shows you where to focus your attention when selecting healthy foods. You want to eat more from the food groups at the base of the pyramid and less from those at the top.

The circle at the center of the pyramid stresses the importance of daily physical activity as part of a healthy eating plan.

and an increased risk of prostate cancer. In a recent study, a high-fat diet increased prostate tumor progression in mice by imitating a gene that encourages cancer growth, which could trigger more aggressive tumors.

However, key questions remain unanswered. It's uncertain whether the relationship between high fat intake and cancer is due to the amount of fat or a specific type of fat. Complicating the analysis is that it's often difficult to distinguish between the effect of fat on cancer development and the effect of calories on cancer risk.

To eat well and prevent disease, including cancer, the key is to find a healthy diet you enjoy and can follow that promotes vegetables and fruits, whole grains, healthy fats, fish and other lean sources of protein, and that limits consumption of red and processed meats, sugar and unhealthy fats. The Mayo Clinic Healthy Weight Pyramid is a good example of a healthy eating plan to improve your overall health.

Vegetables and fruits

Including plenty of vegetables and fruits in your diet may be one of the best things that you can do to improve your health. Fresh vegetables and fruits have a low energy density, meaning there are relatively few calories in a large volume of food. That means that you can eat almost unlimited amounts from these two food groups without worrying about excess calories and increased weight.

In addition to being virtually fat-free and low in calories, vegetables and fruits provide fiber, phytochemicals and a variety of nutrients, including potassium and magnesium, necessary for good health.

Substituting fruits and vegetables for foods that have more fat and calories is a relatively easy way to improve your diet without cutting back on the amount you eat. The key is not to smother your fruits and vegetables with dips or sauces that contain a lot of fat. And limit fruit juice and dried fruits because they're concentrated sources of calories.

Carbohydrates

This group includes a wide range of foods that are a major energy source for your body. Most carbohydrates are plant based. These include grain products such as breads, cereals, rice and pasta. Other food groups providing carbohydrates include starchy vegetables such as potatoes, corn and squash.

When choosing grain products, look for the word *whole* — as in whole wheat — on the packaging. Whole grains contain the bran and the germ, which are sources of fiber, vitamins and minerals such as magnesium. When grains are refined, some of the nutrients and the fiber have been eliminated. As a rule, the less refined a carbohydrate is, the better it is for you.

Carbohydrates are generally low in fat and calories if you choose wisely. Eat plain breads rather than dessert breads, sweet rolls or other baked goods, which are often loaded with sugary ingredients. And be selective about what you add to carbohydrates.

Protein and dairy

Proteins perform many vital roles in cell function. For good health, you should eat some protein every day. However, Americans tend to eat more proteins than needed, exceeding the daily requirement.

This food group contains both plant and animal sources. Plant-based foods rich in protein — and relatively low in fat — include beans, peas and lentils. Animal-based foods rich in protein include meat, poultry, fish and seafood, eggs, and dairy products such as milk, cheese and yogurt. To limit fat and calories, eat fish, poultry without skin, lean meats, and low-fat or fat-free dairy products.

Fats

Many people are surprised to hear fats are important for good health. You need some fat in your diet. How much and the right kinds are important.

Not all fats are equal. Monounsaturated and polyunsaturated fats are healthier fats. Monounsaturated fats include olive oil, canola oil, nuts and nut products, and avocados. Polyunsaturated fats include safflower, corn, sunflower and soy oils, and can be found in varieties of cold-water fish such as salmon. Saturated fats

and trans fats are less healthy. Saturated fats are found in red meat, whole-fat dairy products, butter, lard, coconut oil and other tropical oils. Trans fats are used in commercially produced products such as cookies, pastries, crackers and deep-fried foods.

All fats contain approximately 45 calories per serving and are high-energy-dense foods. For that reason, all fats, even the healthier ones, should be consumed sparingly. One way to cut the fat in your diet is to reduce the amount of butter, margarine and vegetable oil that you add during cooking.

Sweets and alcohol

Cakes, cookies, pastries and other desserts are major sources of calories — mostly from sugar and fat — and they offer little in terms of nutrition. You don't have to give up these foods entirely but be smart about your selections and portion sizes.

Alcohol also provides calories but no nutrients. Regular consumption of alcohol can be unhealthy and often replaces healthier dietary options. If you do drink alcohol, do so in moderation.

PHYSICAL ACTIVITY

It's well known that regular exercise can promote cardiovascular health. When it comes to preventing cancer, the data aren't as clear-cut. However, studies indicate that regular exercise may help reduce cancer risk, including prostate cancer.

Regular exercise has been shown to strengthen your immune system, improve circulation and speed digestion — all of which may play a role in cancer prevention. Exercise also helps prevent obesity, another potential risk factor for some cancers.

In addition, men who are physically active usually develop less severe symptoms of benign prostatic hyperplasia (BPH) than do men who get little exercise. Regular exercise also may help reduce BPH risk.

If you're inactive, it's best to increase your activity gradually. If you're recovering from surgery or another medical treatment, talk with your doctor before beginning an activity program.

Are you fit?

Federal guidelines generally recommend between 30 and 60 minutes of moderate physical activity every day. But, according to a report from the U.S. surgeon general, more than 60% of American adults aren't active on a regular basis and, worse yet, 25% aren't active at all.

Simply put, most Americans aren't physically fit. Being fit allows you to function well in daily life and maintain good health, reducing your risk of many medical conditions. To know if you're fit, consider these indicators:

- You have enough energy to enjoy the activities you want to do.
- You have no problem carrying out the daily tasks of life.
- You can hold a conversation while doing light to moderate exercise.

BEFORE YOU GET STARTED

If you're inactive or have health concerns, it's a good idea to talk with your doctor before starting a physical activity program. If you have another health problem or you're at risk of heart disease, you may need to take special precautions while you exercise.

It's important to see your doctor if you:
- Have blood pressure of 140/90 millimeters of mercury or higher.
- Have diabetes or heart, lung or kidney disease.
- Are age 40 or older and haven't had a recent physical.
- Have a family history of heart-related problems before age 55.
- Are unsure of your health status.
- Have experienced chest discomfort, shortness of breath or dizziness during exercise or strenuous activity.

- You can walk a mile without feeling winded or fatigued.
- You easily climb at least three flights of stairs.

You're probably not as fit as you should be if you feel tired most of the time, you're unable to keep up with others your age, and you become short of breath or fatigued when you walk a short distance.

How to shape up

You can improve your fitness no matter your age and health. However, regular exercise can be a big change if you haven't been active in the recent past.

Many people start an exercise program but don't stick with it — often because they try to do too much too soon. This all-or-nothing mentality is a recipe for discouragement, not to mention possible injury. It's best to start gradually at a pace that you're comfortable with and build from there.

There are different types of exercise, and each benefits your body in a different way. Some exercises are designed to strengthen your heart while others build endurance. Some help keep you flexible while others build bone and muscle mass.

Typically, an exercise program consists of the three major types of exercise: aerobic, flexibility and strength training. Combining regular exercise with a healthy diet can provide you with many health benefits.

Aerobic exercise

Aerobic activities improve cardiovascular fitness — the health of your heart, lungs and circulatory system. This increases your ability to use oxygen, referred to as aerobic capacity. High aerobic capacity gives you more endurance and allows you to work at a more intense level for a longer time. Aerobic exercise burns a lot of calories and can help you lose weight or maintain a healthy weight.

Try to get at least 30 minutes of aerobic exercise on most, if not all, days of the week. But your activity doesn't have to be condensed into one chunk of time — the cumulative effect of physical activity is what matters. If you can't exercise for 30 minutes at a time, aim for at least three 10-minute sessions a day.

Brisk walking is the most common aerobic exercise because it's easy, convenient and inexpensive. All you need is a good pair of walking shoes. Walk at an even, comfortable pace that you can maintain. If you're getting short of breath, slow down.

If brisk walking doesn't appeal to you, you can choose other kinds of aerobic activity. Choose a type of exercise that appeals to you — you're more likely to stick with an exercise program that's fun. Better yet, choose a variety of options! Other forms of aerobic exercise include:
- Bicycling.
- Swimming.
- Jogging.
- Tennis and other racket sports.
- Golfing (when walking, not riding).

- Dancing.
- Basketball.
- Volleyball.
- Water aerobics.
- Cross-country skiing.

Flexibility exercises

Stretching before and after aerobic activity increases the range in which you can bend and stretch your joints, muscles and ligaments. Flexibility exercises also help prevent joint pain and injury.

The stretches should be gentle and slow. Stretch only until you feel slight tension in your muscles. If a stretch hurts, you've gone too far — ease up. If you have time to stretch only once, stretch after your workout because your muscles will be warmed up.

Strength training

When it comes to overall fitness, investing in a set of weights or resistance bands may pay dividends as great as those gained with a pair of walking shoes. Strength training reduces body fat and increases lean muscle mass — allowing you to burn calories more efficiently. The exercises also help improve posture and balance and promote healthy bones.

Strength training involves working your muscles against some form of resistance. When your muscles push or pull against a force such as gravity, a free weight or your own body weight, they gradually grow stronger.

Sessions lasting 20 to 30 minutes two to three times a week are sufficient for most people. Start with five repetitions of each exercise and try to build up to 12 repetitions. Stretch your muscles before and after each workout.

Staying active

About half the people who start an exercise program will drop out within 6 months. Some stop because they get bored or don't see any results. Others overdo exercise and quickly become discouraged by muscle pain and stiffness. The following tips may help you stay motivated and involved.

Be patient

It's better to progress slowly than to push too hard and be forced to abandon your program because of pain or injury. Improvements may not develop overnight, but you'll notice a difference within about a month of regular activity. It generally takes about 3 months for an exercise program to become routine. If you can stay with your program for that long, you're more likely to continue it and enjoy the activity.

Make it fun

Boredom is a major reason why people stop exercising. You're more likely to stick with your program if you take part in activities that you enjoy. Consider working out with a friend or joining a fitness class. Listen to music, watch television or read while you exercise.

Add variety

Alternating between different activities reduces your chance of injury from overusing a muscle or joint. It helps keep all your joints and muscles engaged. It also keeps things more interesting.

Avoid all-or-nothing thinking

On days when time is tight or your motivation is waning, do less, but do something. That said, if you're tired, feel a cold coming on or have a hectic day, don't force yourself to work out.

Get support

Studies show that social support helps people stay with their exercise routines. Committing to exercising with a partner helps you get out the door on those days when you're not inspired. By the same token, if you're signed up for a class, you may be more motivated to attend.

Reward yourself

Work on developing an internal sense of reward based on feelings of accomplishment, self-esteem and self-control. After each activity session, take a few minutes to relax. Savor the good feelings that exercise gives you and reflect on the goals you've just accomplished.

SEEING YOUR DOCTOR REGULARLY

Regular prostate exams also are crucial to good health. If prostate disease does develop, a digital rectal exam or PSA test often can catch the problem in its earliest stages — when the condition is easier to treat. If you don't regularly see a doctor, schedule an appointment to have a general physical exam, and make it a yearly habit.

If you notice prostate-related signs and symptoms — for example, if you experience increased urination, difficulty urinating, pain while urinating, lower pelvic and back pain, or blood in your urine or semen — see your doctor as soon as possible. Even if you believe that it's not a big deal, it's still important to have your symptoms checked out. You don't want to risk the possibility that you could be wrong.

ANSWERS TO YOUR QUESTIONS

Does alcohol play a role in the risk of prostate disease?

There's no evidence that a moderate amount of alcohol causes prostate disease. A moderate amount of alcohol for men is two drinks a day — one drink a day if you're older than age 65.

If you regularly drink more than a moderate amount of alcohol, it may interfere with your diet. People who drink excessive amounts of alcohol often substitute alcohol for food and may not get adequate amounts of nutrients. A poor diet can weaken your immune system and reduce your body's natural defenses against disease. If you drink alcohol, do so in moderation.

Is soy sauce a good source of soy?

No. Soy sauce doesn't contain beneficial amounts of cancer-fighting chemicals, and it's very high in sodium. If you're sensitive to sodium, regular use of soy sauce can increase your blood pressure.

Is it true that stress can cause prostate problems?

It hasn't been proved that stress increases your risk of prostate disease, but there's some evidence that stress may play a role. Stress weakens your immune system, making it more difficult for your body to fight off disease, including cancer. Researchers also theorize that stress can produce tension in your lower pelvic muscles, affecting normal functioning of the prostate gland and, possibly, causing prostatitis.

12

Integrative therapies

As Americans take a more active role in their health care, many are exploring options that are generally not considered part of conventional medical practice. These options include a broad range of healing philosophies, approaches and therapies such as dietary supplements, acupuncture, meditation and Ayurveda, and are referred to collectively as complementary and alternative medicine (CAM). Another commonly used term is integrative medicine.

Integrative medicine describes a change taking place in many health care institutions — integrating CAM therapies with conventional medicine. The goal is to treat the whole person — mind, body and spirit — not just the disease. This is done by combining the best of today's high-tech medicine with the best of nontradi-

tional practices that have high-quality evidence to support their use.

There are legitimate concerns regarding many complementary and alternative products and practices that should be considered before using them. Some therapies still haven't been studied adequately using accepted scientific methods. Often there's conflicting evidence as to whether a treatment actually works — and, if so, how well and for how long. There may also be concerns about quality control, dosage, side effects and negative interactions with other medications you may be taking.

Even so, as young and old alike seek greater control of their own health care, complementary and alternative therapies have become increasingly popular. And a growing body of evidence suggests that some nontraditional therapies may provide some benefits and help you manage your health.

Here's a look at some of the more common complementary and alternative treatments promoted for the prevention or treatment of prostate disease, and for cancer in general.

DIETARY SUPPLEMENTS

As anyone who has walked through a health food store can attest, the profusion of dietary supplements is almost overwhelming. Literally thousands of products crowd the shelves, touting all sorts of claims.

Most dietary supplements are derived from plants or herbs, though minerals, vitamins and even some hormones are included in the category. Supplements — especially the herbal products — are popular because of the perception they're natural and, therefore, good for you.

But being natural doesn't always translate into being safe. Any product that's strong enough to provide a potential benefit to the body can also be strong enough to cause harm. Despite these concerns, certain supplements can be part of your overall wellness plan, provided you use them wisely.

Remember, supplements are just that — supplemental. They can't replace a nutritious diet, regular exercise and adequate sleep.

Prostate concerns

The following herbal products are marketed to relieve common prostate problems — such as frequent urination or weak urine flow.

Pygeum (Pygeum africanum)

An extract from the bark of this tree, also known as the African plum tree, has been shown to improve symptoms of mild to moderate benign prostatic hyperplasia (BPH). Although available as a supplement in the United States, it's more commonly used in European countries.

Pygeum appears to act similarly to 5-alpha reductase inhibitors, regulating muscle tone, although to a much lesser degree. It also has anti-inflammatory properties. The herb has been linked to increased urine flow, more complete urination and reduced need for nighttime urination.

While the herb is generally well tolerated, some people may experience gastrointestinal side effects, including diarrhea, constipation, stomach pain or nausea. More research is needed regarding long-term use.

Beta-sitosterols

Preparations of these naturally occurring plant compounds have been studied as treatments for a number of diseases and conditions. There's some evidence they may improve urinary symptoms of BPH.

There's also some research that suggests in high concentrations, beta-sitosterols may hinder cancer growth and trigger the death of cancer cells. However, more research is needed.

Beta-sitosterols can be found in plant-based foods such as fruits, vegetables, soybeans, breads, peanuts and peanut products. They can be found in sterol-enriched margarines, as well as in supplements.

Saw palmetto

Saw palmetto has become a popular treatment for reducing the symptoms of BPH. In Europe, it's sold as a drug. In the United States, it's available as a dietary supplement in health food stores. It may be sold as a liquid extract, capsules, tablets, or as a tea. Saw palmetto products are made from the berries of this dwarf palm plant, which thrives in the warm climates of southeastern United States.

Some researchers believe saw palmetto affects testosterone, the sex hormone believed to stimulate tissue growth in the prostate gland, although this interaction is still debated. Several studies have suggested saw palmetto may reduce abnormal growth of tissue in the prostate gland.

A 2020 study found evidence that saw palmetto might be as effective as the prescription drug tamsulosin in treating symptoms of BPH, improving such measurements as the International Prostate Symptom Score, maximum flow rate, prostate-specific antigen (PSA) and quality of life.

On the flip side, data sponsored by the National Institutes of Health and the National Center for Complementary and Integrative Health found no significant benefits from taking saw palmetto as compared with a placebo. This isn't to say that the herb isn't effective, but it suggests the need for more research to better understand its benefits.

Saw palmetto is generally safe when used as directed and side effects are rare, but you shouldn't use it if you have a bleeding problem. Most men begin to see improvements in urinary symptoms within 1 to 3 months. If you don't see any benefit after 3 months, the product may not work for you.

Other products

Other herbal products on the market for prostate concerns include:
- African wild potato (*Hypoxis rooperi*), also known as South African star grass.
- Pumpkin seeds (*Cucurbita pepo*).
- Rye grass (*Secale cereale*).
- The above-ground parts of stinging nettle (*Urtica dioica* and *Urtica urens*), also known as common nettle.

If taken in small to moderate amounts, these products appear to be safe. However, they haven't been studied in large, long-term trials to verify their safety or to prove they actually help with prostate symptoms.

Cancer fighters

Several dietary supplements claim to help cure or prevent cancer. There's no scientific evidence that these products can accomplish this, and some of the claims may even be dangerous. A few popular supplements that are sold as cancer-fighting agents are:

Chaparral

Also known as creosote bush or grease-wood, chaparral (*Larrea tridentata*) comes from a desert shrub found in the southwestern United States and Mexico. American Indians used chaparral to treat ailments from the common cold to snakebites.

The herb has been formulated into teas, capsules and tablets, with claims that it can cure a variety of diseases, including cancer. However, studies haven't shown that the herb destroys or prevents cancer, and research suggests it can lead to irreversible liver failure.

Flaxseed

Flaxseed and its oil have been promoted for decades as a supplement with anticancer properties. Past studies indicated that men following a low-fat diet supplemented with flaxseed experienced reduced PSA levels and a reduction in growth rate of prostate cancer cells. But another study found that it was a low-fat diet — not flaxseed — likely responsible for these changes.

Further studies are needed before a clear recommendation can be made. However, flaxseed doesn't appear to cause any harm, and can be a heart-healthy addition to your daily diet. It's important to note that the flaxseed used in research studies was not flaxseed oil. Flaxseed oil may actually cause more harm than good, potentially making prostate tumors more aggressive in some men.

Selenium

As mentioned on page 198, the Selenium and Vitamin E Cancer Prevention Trial (SELECT) for prostate symptoms followed data on men who took one or both of these supplements, compared with those who took a placebo.

While men who took vitamin E alone were shown to have a significant increase in prostate cancer risk, those taking both supplements did not. However, they had no reduction in their prostate cancer risk. Furthermore, men who began the study with high levels of selenium in their bodies showed an increased risk of prostate cancer after taking selenium supplements.

To date, there are no clinical trials that show a clear benefit from taking selenium supplements to prevent prostate cancer.

Shark cartilage

Shark cartilage contains a protein thought to inhibit the formation of new blood vessels in tumors, preventing

Other practices that have received attention as possible cancer fighters include the following:

Chelation therapy. In chelation, a doctor injects a substance into your bloodstream that binds certain molecules so that they can be removed from your system. This is an approved procedure for heavy metal toxicity — removing elements such as lead and mercury — but there's no evidence that chelation can treat other diseases, including cancer. The therapy can produce significant side effects, including kidney and bone marrow damage, an irregular heart rhythm, and severe inflammation of the veins. It should only be performed by a knowledgeable doctor.

Macrobiotics. The philosophy behind macrobiotics is that natural foods, utensils and fabrics, combined with a positive attitude and social interconnectedness, promote health and harmony and fight disease, including cancer. However, there's no evidence that macrobiotics prevents or cures cancer. The diet itself has many health benefits, including being low in fat and high in certain vitamins, minerals and phytochemicals. It may be deficient in other nutrients, though, and may require supplemental nutrients to balance its shortcomings.

cancer in sharks. Therefore, some people believe that capsules containing shark cartilage can do the same in humans — prevent cancer and shrink tumors that have formed. But in limited studies, shark cartilage supplements have generally been shown to be ineffective.

Among other things, it's doubtful that the capsules contain enough purified protein to have an effect. Also, you may digest the protein as you do other proteins, and it may never reach your bloodstream to be of help. In addition to a bad taste, high doses of shark cartilage can cause nausea.

Knowing the risks

Unlike prescription medications, the Food and Drug Administration (FDA) doesn't regulate the effectiveness of dietary supplements. In addition, regulations regarding the safety of these products differ from those of the FDA.

With prescription drugs, the FDA requires that the manufacturer prove that the benefits of the drug outweigh any safety concerns before the drug is approved for sale. With dietary supplements, health officials assume the products are safe until proven otherwise. Only when a supplement is shown to be unsafe is it removed from the market.

The quality and purity of dietary supplements is another challenge. There are numerous reports of altered or impure supplements reaching the market. Fortunately, in 2010, the FDA enacted Good Manufacturing Practices (GMP) standards for all supplements manufactured or sold in the U.S. Basically, the standards require the product to contain exactly what the label claims — nothing more, nothing less.

It's always a good idea to talk to your doctor before you take a dietary supplement. In general, it's wise to avoid dietary supplements if:

- **You're having surgery in the near future.** Supplements may interfere with anesthesia or cause dangerous complications such as bleeding or high blood pressure.
- **You're younger than 18 or older than 65.** Few supplements have been tested on children and adolescents. And older adults may metabolize medications differently than do younger adults taking the same products.
- **You take prescription or nonprescription medications.** Some herbs can cause serious side effects when mixed with certain medications.

MIND-BODY THERAPIES

Mind-body practices are based on the interrelationship of the mind and body, and the power of one to affect the other.

Mind-body therapies are most commonly used to relieve anxiety and stress and to promote an overall sense of well-being. Some evidence shows that they may also strengthen your immune system. Mind-body therapies can't cure prostate disease, but some people find them helpful in coping with the emotional and physical effects of cancer, including pain.

Meditation

Meditation is a way to calm your mind and body. You focus your attention on your breathing or on repetition of a word or sound. This suspends the stream of thoughts that normally occupy your conscious mind, leading to a state of physical relaxation, mental calmness, alertness and psychological balance.

Although meditation may sound simple, learning to control your thoughts isn't easy. The more you practice, though, the easier it gets to concentrate without having your mind wander.

Regular meditation may be used to treat anxiety, stress, pain, depression and insomnia. Studies suggest it may also help reduce blood pressure. The therapy is generally considered safe.

Yoga

The practice of yoga has been around for thousands of years. It involves a series of postures, along with controlled breathing exercises, to help focus your mind more on the moment and less on the concerns of your day. Movement of your body through the poses requires balance and concentration.

Yoga can help reduce stress and anxiety, slow breathing, lower blood pressure, and may also decrease symptoms of back pain. However, to be effective, yoga requires training and regular practice.

Tai chi

Tai chi is sometimes described as meditation in motion. Originally developed in China for self-defense, this graceful form of exercise is becoming increasingly integrated into conventional health care. The benefits of tai chi include stress reduction, increased energy and stamina, and greater balance and flexibility.

Tai chi involves a series of gentle, deliberate postures or movements, with each motion flowing into the next without pause. The practice has virtually no negative side effects.

Massage

The warmth of human touch generally provides comfort and pleasure, and the benefits of massage therapy include relaxation and decreased muscle tension. Massage also may help improve symptoms such as anxiety, pain, fatigue and distress.

Talk with your health care provider about whether massage is safe for you and what areas of your body, if any, a massage

therapist should avoid. Be sure your therapist graduated from an accredited program and meets state licensure requirements.

Humor therapy

Humor therapy is based on the belief that frequent periods of laughter help distract your attention from your health problems. Laughter is also a kind of analgesic — it promotes the release of chemicals that fight pain and reduce depression. Humor therapy simply involves lightening your day by setting aside time to watch a funny movie, attend a comedy show or call a friend who makes you laugh.

Hypnosis

People have been using hypnosis to promote healing since ancient times. The therapy may offer relief to people with disease-related pain, including cancer pain. It's also used in treating stress, anxiety and various behavioral disorders.

Hypnosis produces an induced state of relaxation in which your mind stays focused and open to suggestion. During a session, you receive suggestions designed to increase your ability to cope with your condition. This technique can effectively relieve some chronic pain, and it may also reduce cancer-related nausea and vomiting.

Research indicates that some individuals are more susceptible to hypnotism than are others. Unlike situations sometimes portrayed in movies and on television, you can't be forced under hypnosis to do something that you don't want to do. Since hypnosis poses little risk of harmful side effects, the therapy may be worth a try, if you're interested.

Music, dance and art therapy

One or more of these creative expressions can calm and soothe you, revive your spirits, and in some cases, ease pain and suffering. In addition, they help promote self-confidence and may reduce symptoms of depression.

You don't have to be an accomplished dancer, artist or musician to take part. For example, anyone can listen to and enjoy music. Several national organizations promote the use of music, dance and art for health and healing, with chapters set up across the country.

Animal-assisted therapy

Animal-assisted therapy, also known as pet therapy, is a growing field that uses dogs or other animals to help people recover from or better cope with health problems, including cancer.

A visit with a therapy animal may reduce pain, anxiety, depression and fatigue, all of which are common in people receiving cancer treatment. At Mayo Clinic, certified therapy dogs are part of the Caring Canines Program, making regular hospital visits.

ENERGY THERAPIES

Some integrative therapies center on the belief that natural energy forces play an important role in overall health and healing. When an energy pathway in the body becomes blocked or disturbed, illness results. To heal the body, free flow of energy needs to be restored.

There's no proof that these therapies can treat prostate disease, but they do appear to be safe, and they may provide other health benefits.

Acupuncture

Acupuncture is one of the most studied CAM practices. The National Institutes of Health has issued a consensus statement with evidence that acupuncture helps relieve pain, including certain forms of chronic pain. And clinical studies have shown that acupuncture is effective in reducing pain in some people with cancer. There's stronger evidence that the procedure relieves nausea and vomiting caused by chemotherapy and anesthesia.

During a typical acupuncture session, a practitioner inserts hair-thin needles into your skin in various combinations. The purpose of the needles is to remove blockages and promote the free flow of life energy (chi). The practitioner may gently move the needles or apply electrical stimulation or heat to them.

Inserting the needles should cause little or no pain. Some people even find the procedure relaxing. Adverse side effects from acupuncture are rare but can occur. Make sure your acupuncturist is trained and follows good hygienic practices, including the use of disposable needles.

Acupressure

Acupressure, like acupuncture, stems from the belief that just below your skin are invisible pathways of energy — your body's life forces. During acupressure, a practitioner applies pressure with the fingertips to specific points on your body to restore the free flow of life energy and relieve your symptoms. Research on the benefits of acupressure is inconclusive, but some people find the therapy helpful and relaxing.

OTHER APPROACHES

Some approaches to healing involve complete medical systems based on traditional practices dating back thousands of years. Treatments focus on prevention and restoring a natural balance to enable healing. Studies are limited on the effectiveness of these approaches, and their benefits generally remain unproved.

Ayurveda

This healing philosophy stems from medical practices that originated in India more than 5,000 years ago. Ayurveda is based on the principle that the mind and body are one and that the body cannot be well if the mind is troubled.

Ayurveda practitioners believe that cancer stems from emotional, spiritual and physical imbalances. To treat disease, including cancer, you purge the body of toxic substances through bloodletting, vomiting or emptying the bowels. Diet, breathing exercises and massage help rebuild the proper balance. There's no evidence this practice can cure disease.

Homeopathy

Homeopathic medicine uses highly diluted preparations of natural substances, typically plants and minerals, to treat symptoms of illness. The system is based on a "law of similars." Practitioners believe that if a large dose of a substance causes you to have certain symptoms when you're healthy, a small dose of the same substance can relieve those symptoms.

From a list of nearly 2,000 substances, a homeopath prepares the most appropriate remedy for your set of symptoms. People generally use this approach for conditions such as arthritis, asthma, allergies, colds and influenza. However, scientific research has been unable to confirm that homeopathic medicines work or explain how they might work.

Naturopathy

This system is based on the healing power of nature. It relies on natural remedies such as sunlight, air and water, combined with supplements, to strengthen the body's healing ability.

Much of the advice of naturopaths is worth heeding: Exercise regularly, practice good nutrition, quit smoking and enjoy nature.

However, claims that treatments such as hydrotherapy can detoxify the body and strengthen the immune system aren't backed up by scientific research. And there's no evidence that naturopathy can cure cancer or any other disease, as some proponents claim.

PROTECTING YOURSELF

It's becoming increasingly evident that integrative therapies can play a role in better health. But it's important to remember some of the differences between these nontraditional approaches and more conventional treatments.

If you decide to try complementary and alternative treatments, make sure to protect your health — and your wallet

TOO GOOD TO BE TRUE?

The Food and Drug Administration and the National Council Against Health Fraud recommend that you watch for use of the following practices. These are often warning signs of potentially fraudulent products or therapies:

- The advertisements or promotional materials include words such as breakthrough, magical or new discovery. If the product or therapy were in fact a cure, it would be widely reported in the media and your doctor would recommend its use.
- The product materials include pseudo-medical jargon such as detoxify, purify or energize. Such descriptions are difficult to define and measure.
- The manufacturer claims the product can treat a wide range of symptoms, or cure or prevent several diseases. No single product can do this.
- The product seems to be backed by scientific studies, but references for the research studies aren't provided, are very limited or are out of date. Manufacturers of legitimate products like to promote the results of scientific studies, not hide them. Also use caution with any treatment not available or approved for use in the United States or Europe. You can find FDA-approved drugs by entering Drugs@FDA into your web browser.
- The product has no negative side effects, only benefits. Most medications and other therapies have some side effects.
- The manufacturer accuses the government, medical profession or drug companies of suppressing important information about the helpfulness of the product. There's no reason for the government or medical profession to do so.

— by learning all you can about the treatments and what benefits their practitioners claim they provide.

The National Center for Complementary and Integrative Health (NCCIH) recommends the following steps:

Research its safety and effectiveness

The benefits you receive from a treatment should outweigh its risks. To find out more about a therapy, check the scientific literature. You also can request information from the NCCIH or visit their website (see page 220). Be aware that many websites that tout health information are merely advertising fronts for various products.

Check out the practitioner or manufacturer

If you're working with a licensed practitioner, check with your local and state medical boards for information about the person's credentials and whether any complaints have been filed against that person. If you're buying a product from a business, check with your local or state business bureau to find out whether any complaints have been filed against the company.

Estimate the total cost

Because many complementary and alternative approaches aren't covered by health insurance, it's important to know exactly how much the treatment will cost you.

Talk with your doctor

Your health care provider can help you determine whether the treatment may be beneficial and if it's safe. Some complementary and alternative therapies may interfere with medications you're taking or adversely affect other health conditions you have.

Don't substitute proven for unproven

If it's been proved that medication, surgery or another treatment recommended by your doctor can help your condition, don't replace this treatment with alternative products, practices or therapies that haven't been proved effective.

TAKING RESPONSIBILITY

Good health doesn't just happen. It generally stems from wise decisions you make, such as avoiding smoking, limiting alcohol use, controlling stress and practicing other healthy habits.

It's true that there are some factors related to prostate health that you have no control over or can't change. But when changes or concerns develop you can act on them. Seeing a doctor promptly and having a prostate examination increase your chances of identifying prostate problems early — when it's more likely they can be treated and cured.

The choices you make day in and day out can keep your prostate healthy — or help it to become healthy again. This may require lifestyle changes, such as eating a more nutritious diet and increasing your level of physical activity. Discuss complementary and alternative therapies with your doctor to reduce the risk of potentially dangerous side effects from questionable products or practices.

It's all about taking responsibility for your own well-being. The fact that you're reading this book is an important first step in this process, and an indication that you want to make the right decisions for treating or preventing prostate disease.

Additional resources

Contact these organizations for more on prostate health, including information about prostatitis, benign prostatic hyperplasia and prostate cancer.

American Cancer Society
www.cancer.org

American College of Radiology
www.acr.org

American Institute for Cancer Research
www.aicr.org

American Urological Association
www.auanet.org

CancerCare
www.cancercare.org

Cancer Research Institute
www.cancerresearch.org

Centers for Disease Control and Prevention
www.cdc.gov

Mayo Clinic
www.MayoClinic.org

National Association for Continence
www.nafc.org

National Cancer Institute
www.cancer.gov

National Center for Complementary and Integrative Health
www.nccih.nih.gov

National Coalition for Cancer Survivorship
www.canceradvocacy.org

National Comprehensive Cancer Network
www.nccn.org

National Institutes of Health
Clinical Trials
www.clinicaltrials.gov

Natural Medicines Comprehensive Database
www.naturaldatabase.com

Prostate Cancer Foundation
www.pcf.org

Radiological Society of North America
www.rsna.org

Urology Care Foundation
www.urologyhealth.org

ZERO: The End of Prostate Cancer
www.zerocancer.org

Glossary

A

ablation. The removal or destruction of a body part or tissue or its function.

active surveillance. The decision to hold off on aggressive treatment and observe your condition to see if it changes.

androgen. A hormone, such as testosterone, that is responsible for the development of male sex organs and other male features, such as facial hair and musculature.

antiandrogen therapy. Medications that prevent the testosterone produced in adrenal glands from reaching prostate cancer cells.

anticholinergic drug. A medication that relaxes the muscles of an overactive bladder, helping control symptoms of BPH.

antioxidant. A substance found in many vegetables and fruits that may protect body cells from the damaging effects of free radicals, substances that may cause cancer.

apoptosis. Programmed cell death, which helps keep normal cell growth balanced and destroys abnormal cells. In cancer cells, this mechanism is disrupted, and the cells live longer than normal and grow without restraint.

B

benign prostatic hyperplasia (BPH). A noncancerous condition that results when tissue in the interior of the prostate gland enlarges and presses on the urethra, narrowing the channel and restricting the normal flow of urine.

biomarker. A distinctive, measurable biological indicator of a condition, such as cancer.

biopsy. A standard diagnostic procedure in which a doctor removes a tiny sample of tissue from your body. The sample is examined under a microscope for signs of disease, such as cancer.

bladder. A hollow, expandable organ in your pelvic region that stores urine, which is produced in the kidneys and transported to the bladder via the ureters. Urine exits the bladder through the urethra.

bone scan. A nuclear imaging procedure based on a radioactive solution that's been injected into your bloodstream. The solution migrates to areas of bone activity that may stem from cancer.

brachytherapy. A treatment for prostate cancer that involves implanting small radioactive seeds directly in or near the prostate gland. The implantation may be permanent or temporary.

bulking agent. A substance injected into the urethra that puffs up urethral tissue and narrows the opening of your bladder. Bulking agents are used to treat incontinence.

C

catheter. A thin, flexible tube that can be inserted into your body to inject or drain fluid. A catheter inserted through the penis and urethra allows urine to drain from the bladder.

chemotherapy. A treatment for prostate cancer that uses chemicals to destroy the cancer cells. Unfortunately, the chemicals can attack healthy cells as well, causing side effects.

chronic pelvic pain. A form of prostatitis with symptoms that involve more than just the prostate and are spread throughout the entire pelvic region. This syndrome is difficult to treat because the cause or causes of the pain are unclear.

clinical staging. A series of tests that are done to discover the full extent of cancer in your body — both at its site of origin and its spread to other parts of the body. Also called staging.

complementary and alternative therapies. A broad range of healing philosophies, approaches and techniques that often lie outside conventional medical practice. Also known as integrative medicine.

computerized tomography (CT). A procedure that uses X-rays to create cross-sectional images of your body's interior with a greater degree of detail and clarity than standard X-rays can provide. A CT scan can locate prostate infections, obstructions and cancer.

cryoablation. A procedure in which a doctor inserts freezing probes into an organ, such as the prostate gland. Argon gas is used to freeze and kill the abnormal cells. Also called cryotherapy or freeze therapy.

cystitis. Inflammation of the bladder, often due to infection. Cystitis can lead to painful urination.

cystoscopy. A procedure that uses a flexible tube, equipped with a lens and a light, that is threaded into your body. The procedure provides clear images of the urethra and bladder that may help your doctor understand what's obstructing your urine flow.

D

digital rectal examination (DRE). A diagnostic procedure in which a doctor inserts a gloved finger into your rectum to feel the prostate gland. A prostate that feels abnormal to the touch may indicate an infection, enlargement or cancer.

dysuria. A painful, burning discharge of urine, often as a result of inflammation or infection in the bladder.

E

ejaculation. The release of semen through the penis that occurs during male orgasm. This function may be affected by prostate problems or may be a side effect of treatment.

erectile dysfunction. The inability to maintain a firm erection during intercourse. This may be a problem when pelvic nerves are damaged during surgery, radiation therapy or cryotherapy. Sometimes called impotence.

estrogen. A hormone, produced primarily in females but also in males, that helps the body develop feminine physical characteristics. As a medication for prostate cancer, estrogen may be used to block the activity of testosterone.

external beam radiotherapy (EBRT). A procedure that directs a concentrated beam of high-energy radiation from a device outside your body to kill cancer cells at specific locations in the body.

F

focal therapy. A therapy that's designed to precisely target areas for treatment, preserving as much unaffected tissue as possible. Focal therapy uses extremely high or extremely low temperatures to destroy very specific areas of tissue

(ablation). Several therapies fall within this category.

G

Gleason grading scale. A system to describe the aggressiveness of a tumor that's been biopsied, named for its creator, Donald Gleason, M.D. The Gleason scale goes from 1 to 5, with 1 being the least aggressive form of cancer.

gynecomastia. Excessive growth of male breasts due to lack of the sex hormone testosterone. This is sometimes a side effect of androgen-deprivation therapy.

H

heat therapy (thermotherapy). Treatments for BPH that use computer-controlled heat to destroy excess prostate tissue. Different forms use microwaves, high-frequency radio waves and lasers.

hematospermia. The presence of blood in semen.

hematuria. The presence of blood in urine.

hormone. A chemical messenger secreted by one of the endocrine glands and carried through the bloodstream. Hormones help regulate many body functions, including digestion, metabolism and reproduction. They may play a role in prostate cancer development.

hormone therapy. Treatment with drugs or surgery that reduces the supply of male sex hormones such as testosterone, which can stimulate prostate cancer cells. Another form of this treatment blocks hormones from reaching the cancer. Also called hormone deprivation therapy or androgen-deprivation therapy.

I

impotence. The inability to maintain a firm erection during sexual intercourse. See erectile dysfunction.

incontinence (urinary). The inability to control the release of urine, which often may be a temporary side effect of prostate treatment.

indolent. Describes the stage of a disease, such as cancer, when it develops slowly and produces few symptoms.

international prostate symptoms score (IPSS). A series of standardized questions that help you and your doctor determine how prostate symptoms are affecting you and guide decisions on how you should be treated.

intravenous pyelogram. An X-ray procedure that uses contrast dye to detect urinary obstructions.

K

Kegel exercises. Voluntary movements of your pelvic floor muscles to improve their strength and tone. Kegel exercises can help reduce mild to moderate incontinence.

L

laparoscopy. Surgery to examine the inside of your abdomen with a laparoscope and remove lymph nodes from your pelvic area suspected of being cancerous. A laparoscope is a thin, lighted tube containing a fiberoptic camera.

latent. Describes the stage of a disease, such as cancer, when it is present in your body but inactive, producing no symptoms.

LH-RH agonist. A medication for prostate cancer that interrupts the activity of the LH-RH hormone (see next entry). As a result, your testicles never get the message to produce testosterone.

luteinizing hormone-releasing hormone (LH-RH). A hormone that alerts the pituitary gland to release luteinizing hormone (LH). In turn, LH signals your testicles to make testosterone, which stimulates prostate cancer cells.

lymph node biopsy. A procedure to remove tissue from the lymph nodes so that the samples can be examined for signs of cancer.

lymph nodes. Small, bean-shaped structures located throughout your body that are critical to your immune system. They store special cells that help protect you from bacteria and other organisms.

M

magnetic resonance imaging (MRI). Imaging procedure that uses magnetic fields to produce detailed pictures of your body's interior.

maximum androgen blockade. Treatment designed to stop your body from producing male hormones. This treatment can include hormone medications, surgery to remove the testicles, or both.

metastasis. The spread of disease-producing agents, such as cancer or bacteria, from one location in the body to another location.

metastatic prostate cancer. Abnormal cell growth that has spread outside the prostate gland to tissue in the lymph nodes, bones and other organs in your body.

mutation. A change or alteration in cell DNA. Sometimes, this change has no effect or can improve the organism, and other times it can hurt the organism.

N

needle biopsy. A procedure in which a surgeon inserts a small needle into an organ, such as the prostate gland. Using the needle, the surgeon removes tiny samples of tissue, which are examined in a laboratory for signs of cancer.

O

open prostatectomy. Surgery to remove internal tissue of the prostate that's obstructing the urethra. The procedure also may be used to relieve severe symptoms of BPH.

orchiectomy. Surgery to remove the testicles, which prevents the production of testosterone. Hormone-blocking drugs have reduced the need for this form of surgery. Also called castration.

P

palpable tumor. An abnormal growth of tissue that can be felt (palpated) — for example, during a digital rectal examination.

pelvic floor muscles. A layer of strong muscle tissue in the lower part of your pelvis that helps control bladder function and bowel movements.

pelvic lymph node dissection. A procedure to remove lymph nodes located near the prostate gland. A pathologist will examine the tissue in a laboratory to discover whether cancer has spread.

perineal prostatectomy. A procedure in which a surgeon makes an incision in the perineum to remove the prostate gland. The perineum is the space between the scrotum and the anus.

peripheral zone. One of the zones of the prostate located on the outer edge of the organ. Very often if there's prostate cancer, it will develop first in the peripheral zone.

positron emission tomography (PET). A form of imaging that uses a radioactive tracer to measure the chemical processes taking place in your body. It's used to detect the presence of cancer.

proctitis. An inflamed rectum, often occurring with bleeding, diarrhea and pain.

prostate gland. An organ that's located just below a man's bladder and surrounds the top of the urethra. This gland produces most of the fluids in semen.

prostate-specific antigen (PSA). A protein produced by the prostate gland that's a vital component of semen. A PSA test can determine how much of this protein is circulating in your blood. PSA comes in two forms — that which is bound to blood proteins, and that which is unbound, called free PSA.

prostatic intraepithelial neoplasia (PIN). Abnormal prostate cells found in biopsies that may signal an increased chance that cancer will develop. PIN samples are usually classified as high grade, indicating the level of risk.

prostatic stent. A tiny metal coil that is inserted into the urethra. When in place, the stent expands to widen the urethra and keep it open.

prostatitis. A general term for inflammation of the prostate gland. The condition encompasses four distinct categories.

proton beam therapy. A form of external beam radiotherapy that uses the positively charged parts of an atom (protons) instead of X-rays to destroy cancer.

R

radiation oncologist. A specialist in cancer treatment who performs radiation therapy.

radiation therapy. The use of radiation — with either an external beam or internal implants or seeds — to kill cancer cells.

radical prostatectomy. A procedure in which a surgeon removes your entire prostate gland, usually along with nearby tissue. Depending on where the incision is made, the surgery may be retropubic (in the lower abdomen) or perineal (between the anus and scrotum).

radioactive seed implant. See brachytherapy.

rectum. The final section of the large intestine, which stores solid waste before it's eliminated. A doctor feels the inner wall of your rectum, which lies next to the prostate, to check for tumors and other abnormalities.

recurrence. A return of cancer after treatment. The recurrence may mean that some cancer cells remained in the body after cancer treatment, or a new cancer may have formed.

resectoscope. A thin, tubular device containing a sliding knife or electrified wire, which can be used for certain surgical procedures of the prostate.

robot-assisted laparoscopic radical prostatectomy (RALRP). A surgical procedure for prostate cancer in which all instruments are controlled by a mechanical device that's guided by a surgeon using a computer console, based on the principles of laparoscopic surgery.

S

semen. A thick, whitish fluid containing sperm cells. Men discharge this fluid from the penis during ejaculation.

seminal vesicles. Saclike glands located behind the bladder that store and produce most of the ejaculatory fluid in semen. Removal of these structures may occur during prostate cancer treatment.

sperm. Male reproductive cells that are produced in the testicles and transmitted in semen.

sphincter. A ring of muscle fiber that opens and contracts to control the release of urine from the bladder. An internal sphincter encircles the bladder opening to the urethra, and an external sphincter is located just below the prostate.

staging. *See clinical staging.*

surgical margins. The borders of tissue that are cut and removed during surgery. One goal of prostate cancer surgery is to remove the prostate gland in a way that leaves behind tissue edges (margins) that are free of cancer.

T

testicles. The egg-shaped glands in the scrotum that produce sperm as well as testosterone.

testosterone. A sex hormone manufactured in the testicles that produces male sexual characteristics. This hormone is an androgen that can stimulate the growth of prostate cancer.

TNM system. A method for describing the spread of cancer. T stands for tumor and signifies the extent of the cancer in, and adjacent to, the prostate gland. N stands for nodes and signifies whether the cancer has spread to nearby lymph nodes. M stands for metastasis — cancer that has spread to other tissues or organs.

transitional zone. One of the zones of the prostate gland. This internal zone surrounds the urethra and is often the part of the prostate that enlarges in older men to cause BPH.

transrectal ultrasound. An imaging technique that uses sound waves, which are bounced off the prostate gland and converted into an image of the prostate and surrounding tissues.

transurethral incision of the prostate (TUIP). A procedure in which a surgeon makes several small incisions in the prostate gland and bladder neck. These cuts allow the urethra to expand, making it easier to urinate.

transurethral microwave thermotherapy (TUMT). A form of heat therapy that uses microwave energy to destroy internal tissue in an enlarged prostate gland that may be obstructing the urethra.

transurethral resection of the prostate (TURP). A procedure in which a surgeon threads a resectoscope into the urethra and cuts away excess prostate tissue. TURP has the longest history of successful relief of BPH symptoms in men with enlarged prostate glands or the most bothersome symptoms.

tumor. An abnormal growth of tissue. The growth may be cancerous (malignant) or noncancerous (benign).

tumor markers. Substances circulating in the blood that are produced by tumors. The amount of a tumor marker in circulation may reflect the extent of the tumor.

U

ultrasonography. An imaging technique that uses the echoes of sound waves directed into the body to create an image of its internal structures. A transrectal ultrasound is frequently used for diagnosing prostate problems.

ureters. The tubes that carry urine from your kidneys to your bladder.

urethra. The tube extending from the bladder to the tip of the penis. The urethra carries urine from the bladder. During ejaculation, the urethra also transports semen from the prostate.

urodynamic studies. A series of tests that helps a doctor assess bladder function.

urologist. A doctor who specializes in treating disorders of the urinary and reproductive systems in men.

V

vasa deferentia. Two tubes that carry sperm from the testicles to the prostate gland and urethra. These will be severed during a prostatectomy.

voiding diary. A means of tracking fluid intake and urination habits to help assess BPH.

Index

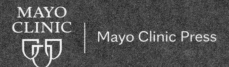
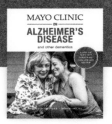
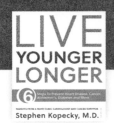
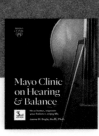
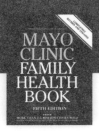
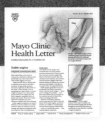